THE GAME OF EATING SMART

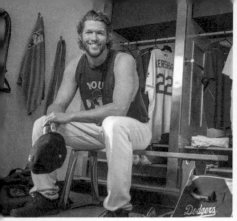
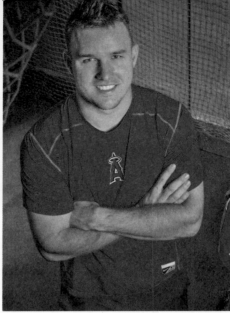
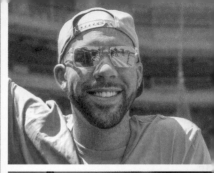
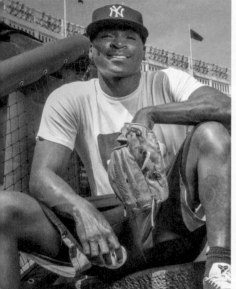
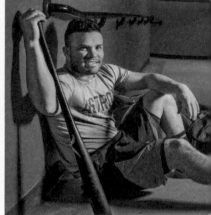
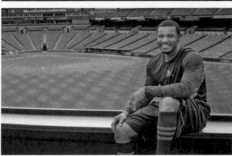
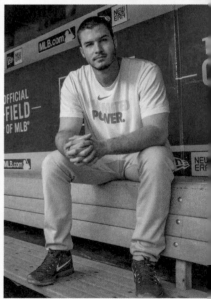
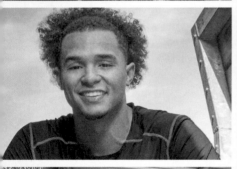
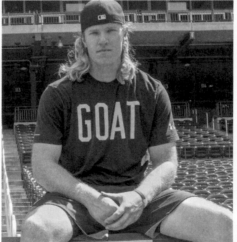
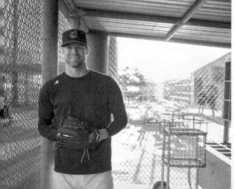
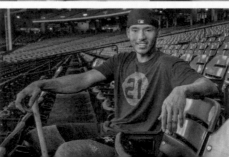
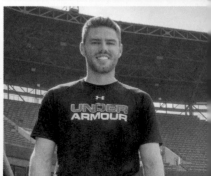

THE GAME OF EATING SMART

*Nourishing Recipes for
Peak Performance Inspired
by MLB® Superstars*

Julie Loria

with Chef Allen Campbell

Photographs by Ben Fink

RODALE
NEW YORK

In memory of José Fernandez, 1992–2016

Published in the United States by Rodale
Books, an imprint of the Crown Publishing
Group, a division of Penguin Random House LLC,
New York.
crownpublishing.com
rodalebooks.com

RODALE and the Plant colophon are registered
trademarks of Penguin Random House LLC.

Major League Baseball players used with
permission of the Major League Baseball
Players Association.
Major League Baseball trademarks and
copyrights are used with permission of Major
League Baseball Properties, Inc.

Library of Congress Cataloging-in-Publication
Data is available upon request.

ISBN 978-1-63565-270-3
Ebook ISBN 978-1-63565-271-3

Printed in China

Book and cover design by Ian Dingman
Interior and cover photographs by Ben Fink
Additional photography credits: pages 142-43
(Matt Kemp) by Rob Leiter/MLB Photos; pages
184-85 (Hunter Pence) by Brad Mangin/MLB
Photos; page 240 (Julie Loria) by Ben Fink;
(Allen Campbell) by Vanessa Flores

10 9 8 7 6 5 4 3 2 1

First Edition

Contents

Introduction **6**

COOKING TIPS AND TECHNIQUES FOR EATING SMART

THE LINEUP AND GAME-CHANGING RECIPES

INTRODUCTION

A box of doughnuts sits untouched in plain sight on a table outside the Houston Astros Spring Training clubhouse. It is 8:00 a.m., and I'm about to interview José Altuve. Soon after that, I'll talk with his teammate Carlos Correa. I can't help but notice that the indulgent breakfast sweets do not tempt either megastar. When it comes to clubhouse cravings, baseball players these days reach for fruits and vegetables, not pastries and other highly processed foods.

But that change is just the beginning. In Major League Baseball, the transition to eating healthy food has become more than a movement; it's a revolution. Players have learned that proper nutrition has a positive impact on athletic performance. Their superfit physiques are like high-end sports cars. And much like Ferrari owners, professional baseball players know not to put low-octane gas into their tanks if they want their finely tuned engines to run well. They now know it's vital to fuel themselves with food that boosts energy and, in turn, confidence. These players credit their improved eating habits with fewer aches, pains, and injuries, faster muscle recovery, better focus on the field—and, in some cases, longer careers.

When I became aware of the lifestyle changes these players have undertaken, I knew I needed to share their insider know-how. Traveling around the country to interview today's elite players was a significant part of my journey toward writing this book. Many of them candidly revealed their personal views on nutrition. They talked openly with me about their eating habits during the season and in the off-season. Some players avoid gluten and dairy altogether. Some prefer plant-based meals and have greatly reduced their red meat intake. Many have cut back on refined sugar, and nearly all of them emphasized the importance of staying hydrated.

Visiting Major League and Spring Training clubhouse kitchens was also an eye-opener. I saw firsthand how much the food scene has changed in professional baseball since I first set foot in a clubhouse more than ten years ago. For too long, doughnuts and other nutrient-free foods were the favored fare. But in the last few years, the seismic shift toward eating nourishing food has become the new normal.

Nearly all of the thirty MLB teams have moved toward serving healthy food and emphasizing a nutritional eating plan. Many of the clubhouses are newly equipped with fresh juice bars and smoothie stations. High-tech appliances are in place to enable the preparation of turmeric and wheatgrass shots. Shelves are stocked with almond and coconut milks, protein powders and superfoods, and side-by-side dispensers full of raw organic nuts and seeds for on-the-go snacks. Jars of coconut oil and shakers of Himalayan pink salt are on hand. And all this just scratches the surface of this food revolution.

That said, top athletes are only human.

Though very mindful of the food they eat, now and then, these players still enjoy an occasional slice of pizza, a scoop of ice cream, or maybe even a doughnut. But you can be certain that such indulgences are now the exception, not the rule. When it comes to what they eat, the goal of today's top baseball players is not perfection, but to make healthy choices more often than not.

It's relatively simple to crave nutrient-dense whole foods when you start to feel and look amazing. The twenty-one star ballplayers featured in this book are living proof of the positive effect of keeping your body fueled the right way. That doesn't mean calorie-counting and fad diets. It simply means consuming more nourishing food—including leafy greens, lean protein, and fresh fruit—that eventually decreases the desire to make unhealthy choices. Of course, you don't have to be a professional athlete to notice the benefits of eating right. The healthy food movement is all around us, and with these simple and nourishing recipes, you too can get into the game of eating smart.

—*Julie Loria*

Teaming Up with Chef Allen Campbell

After I finished all of my interviews, I wanted to develop recipes that reflected the healthy-food philosophies of each of the Major League Baseball players who spoke with me. I wanted to be sure every dish was expertly and carefully created based on what they liked to eat. To help accomplish that goal, I sought out Chef Allen Campbell.

Like Allen, I am Massachusetts-born, and like most natives, I was raised with a passion for Boston sports teams. And though it has been twenty years since I lived in New England, I was very familiar with Allen's work promoting health and wellness for elite athletes in the region: His reputation preceded him. For three years he was the personal chef for New England Patriots' star quarterback Tom Brady and his supermodel wife, Gisele Bündchen.

Together we have teamed up to share more than 100 nutritious and mouthwatering recipes inspired by the palates of twenty-one elite athletes. These include several plant-based dishes along with fish and meat recipes. Many of the players I spoke with try to eat wild-caught fish and grass-fed beef whenever possible. They also try to minimize inflammation as much as they can, so all of the recipes are free of dairy and gluten, which can exacerbate swelling throughout the body. Nor do these recipes include any refined sugar.

Both Allen and I believe that we can make a difference in the health of current and future generations by providing you with the knowledge to make nourishing food that fuels mind and body. What's more, we want to show you just how flavorful healthy food can be.

COOKING TIPS AND TECHNIQUES FOR EATING SMART

Stock Your Kitchen

A well-stocked kitchen is an essential time saver for planning meals. Listed below are key ingredients for making the recipes in this cookbook. Since all of the recipes here are gluten- and dairy-free, you will not find any wheat or dairy products among these lists. And when at all possible, organic choices are best.

Spices

Allspice
Black peppercorns
Cayenne
Chili powder
Crushed red pepper
    flakes
Dried oregano
Dried sage
Ground cinnamon
Ground cloves
Ground coriander
Ground cumin
Ground ginger root
Ground nutmeg
Ground turmeric root
Old Bay seasoning
Smoked paprika

Beans

Black beans
Cannellini beans (aka
    white beans)
Chickpeas (aka garbanzo
    beans)
Kidney beans
Lentils
Mung beans

Grains

Brown basmati rice
Millet
Quinoa (technically this is
    a seed, not a grain)
Short-grain brown rice

Nuts
(raw is best)

Almonds

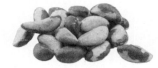

Brazil nuts ▲
Cashews
Pecans
Pistachios
Walnuts

Seeds
(raw is best; refrigerate after opening)

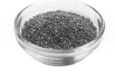

Chia seeds ▲
Hemp hearts (shelled
    hemp seeds)
Pumpkin seeds
Sesame seeds
Sunflower seeds
Whole flaxseeds

Cooking Oils

Avocado oil
Coconut oil (this is the
    preferred oil for recipes
    throughout the book)

Finishing Oils

Extra-virgin olive oil
Nut oils (such as walnut or
    almond)
Sesame oil (toasted and
    untoasted)

Vinegars and Condiments

Champagne vinegar
Cider vinegar
Nutritional yeast (an
    inactive yeast with a

nutty, cheesy flavor and a great nondairy/vegan alternative to Parmesan cheese)
Red wine vinegar
Rice wine vinegar
Sherry vinegar
Tamari (gluten-free soy sauce)
White wine vinegar

Salt

Salt (unrefined salts like sea salt, Himalayan salt and kosher salt are preferred throughout the book)
Smoked salt

Sweeteners

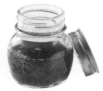

Coconut nectar ▲
Coconut sugar
Pure maple syrup
Raw honey

Flours and Other Baking Ingredients

Almond meal/flour
Baking powder

Brown rice flour
Coconut flour
Garbanzo flour
Oat flour
Rolled oats

Steel-cut oats ▲
Unsweetened coconut flakes
Unsweetened shredded coconut
Vanilla extract

Refrigerator Staples

Hydration:

Aloe water
Coconut water (high-pressure processing (HPP) organic brands are best and are found in the refrigerated section of most grocers)
Filtered water

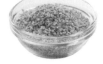

Lemons ▲

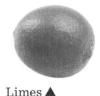

Limes ▲

Condiments:

Organic ketchup
Mustard (yellow or stoneground)

Miscellaneous

Almond butter (and other nut butters such as pecan or walnut)
Avocados
Carrots
Eggs
Garlic
Ginger (fresh ginger root)

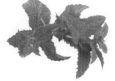

Mint (fresh leaves) ▲
Nut milks (learn how to make your own on page 13)
Onions
Sweet Potatoes

Kitchen Essentials

Equipping your kitchen with useful cookware, tools, and appliances is helpful preparation for making most meals, drinks, and smoothies. Here are some basics that should be within reach.

- Baking dishes (rectangular small, medium, and large in ceramic or glass)
- Baking sheets (stainless steel)
- Baking mat (nonstick silicone)
- Blender (2–3 horsepower, 1500–1800 watts)
- Box grater
- Cast-iron skillet
- Coffee grinder (a small portable one is ideal for grinding whole flaxseed or fresh herbs)
- Cutting boards
- Food processor
- Knife set (chef, slicer, serrated, paring, cleaver, and sharpening steel)
- Juicer (a high-speed centrifugal juicer is the most common type; a masticating juicer is slower and less heat-producing, and is good for leafy greens)
- Mandoline
- Measuring cups
- Measuring spoons
- Microplane
- Mixing bowls (2 cup to 5 quart)
- Muffin tins
- Nut-milk bag (essential if you are going to make your own nut milk)
- Peeler
- Peppermill (for grinding whole peppercorns)
- Pots and pans (small, medium, and large stainless steel saucepans and non-PFOA/PTFE nonstick skillets)
- Salad spinner
- Scoops: #60 (.56 ounce) and #100 (.37 ounce)
- Spatulas (offset and regular)
- Steamer basket
- Strainer (fine-mesh)
- Wax paper for baking and wrapping food (preferably nonbleached)
- Whisks

Soaking and Cooking Beans and Grains

NOTE: Soaking beans and grains in water with cider vinegar makes them easier to digest and makes their nutrients more readily absorbable. The longer they soak, the more beneficial for digestion.

SOAKING BEANS AND LENTILS: In a large pot, bring 8 cups water and 1 tablespoon cider vinegar to a boil for 1 to 2 minutes. Remove from the heat and add 1 cup dry beans or lentils. Soak overnight, uncovered. Strain through a fine-mesh strainer and rinse with cold water. Drain well.

SOAKING RICE, QUINOA, AND MILLET: In a deep bowl, preferably glass, combine $^{2}/_{3}$ cup rice (or quinoa or millet) in room-temperature water to come 4 inches above the rice (or quinoa or millet) and a couple drops of cider vinegar. Soak for at least $1^{1}/_{2}$ hours and as long as 12 hours. Strain through a fine-mesh strainer and rinse with cold water. Drain well.

CANNELLINI BEANS/CHICKPEAS/ KIDNEY BEANS/BLACK BEANS

Makes 2 to 3 cups

1. In a large pot, combine 6 cups water and 1 cup of beans.

2. Over medium-low heat, bring the beans to a gentle simmer and cook, covered, adding water as needed, for 2 to 4 hours, until tender, stirring occasionally. Ccooking time for black beans and chickpeas is 3½ to 4 hours; cooking time for cannellini beans and kidney beans is 2½ to 3 hours.

FRENCH LENTILS/BLACK LENTILS/ MUNG BEANS

Makes 2 to 3 cups

1. In a large saucepan, combine 3 cups water and 1 cup lentils or mung beans.

2. Over medium-low heat, bring the lentils or beans to a gentle simmer and cook, covered, for 25 to 30 minutes, until tender, stirring occasionally.

GREEN LENTILS

Makes 2 to 3 cups

1. In a large saucepan, combine 3 cups water and 1 cup lentils.

2. Over medium-low heat, bring the lentils to a gentle simmer and cook, covered, for 20 to 25 minutes, until tender.

SHORT-GRAIN BROWN RICE

Makes 2 cups

1. In a small saucepan, combine ⅔ cup rice to 1⅓ cups water.

2. Over medium-low heat, bring to a gentle simmer and cook, covered, for 14 to 18 minutes, until tender.

QUINOA AND MILLET

Makes 2 cups

1. In a small saucepan, combine ⅔ cup of quinoa or millet to 1⅓ cups water.

2. Over medium-low heat, bring to a gentle simmer and cook, covered, until the grains are tender. Cooking time for quinoa is 14 to 16 minutes; cooking time for millet is 12 to 14 minutes.

NOTE: Soaking grains decreases cooking times.

Homemade Nut Milks

NOTE: For a consistency similar to that of whole milk, use 1½ cups almonds or shredded coconut. For a thicker consistency, increase the nuts or coconut flakes to 2 cups. In place of almonds, you can use almost any nut to make nut milk, such as cashews, brazil nuts, macadamia nuts, pecans, and walnuts. If using cashews, they do not have to be strained (step 2) since they blend smooth.

ALMOND/COCONUT MILK

Makes 7 cups

1½ to 2 cups almonds or unsweetened shredded coconut

6 cups cold water (add more water for a thinner consistency)

For sweetened milk, add the following:

2 pitted dates

1 teaspoon vanilla extract

Pinch of ground cinnamon, nutmeg, or cloves

1. In a high-powered blender, process all of the ingredients for 2 minutes.

2. Strain through a nut-milk bag and refrigerate in an airtight container. The milk will keep for about 5 days.

THE LINEUP AND GAME-CHANGING RECIPES

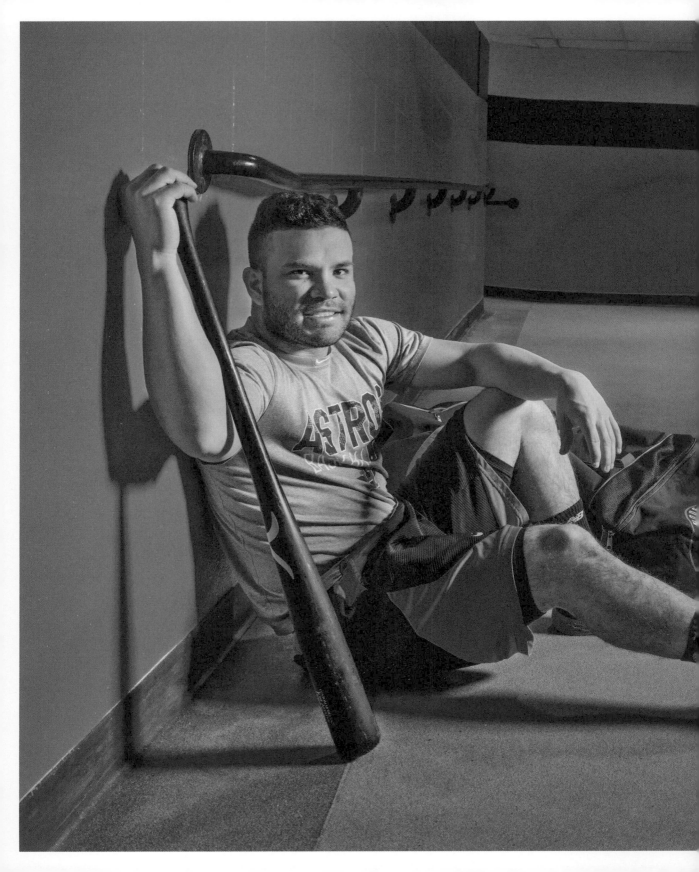

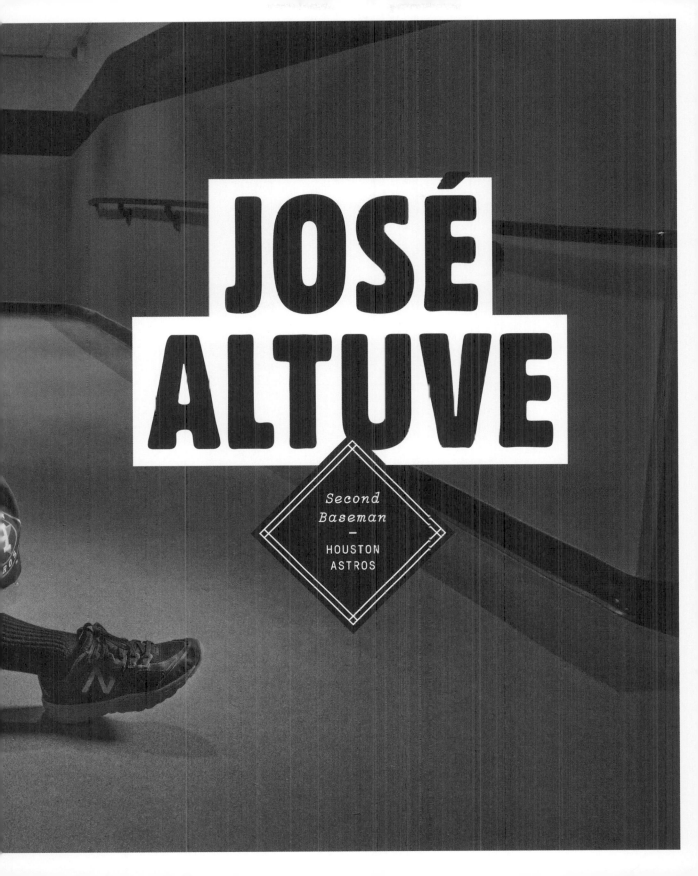

JOSÉ ALTUVE

Second Baseman

—

HOUSTON
ASTROS

My motivation for eating smart comes from my family. We are a healthy family that likes to eat right. Also, my dad noticed some of the big league players eating well and playing well, so he recommended that I improve my diet. Since I changed my diet a few years ago, I've noticed a big difference in my performance.

I've noticed a connection between my eating habits and performance because when I eat right, I not only go out there and play well, I also feel well. I feel better on and off the field, and my recovery is much faster. Once I started eating better, I noticed a 100 percent change. Now I can play all season and I still feel great after it's over. After the season, I still want to go out there and play baseball. I feel faster, and after a game I sleep better. I feel very healthy.

My breakfast routine starts at about 7:00 a.m. with an omelet of spinach, onions, and tomatoes and two pieces of wheat bread. I eat some fruit too, usually pineapple. I also eat bananas and watermelon, and occasionally an apple. I like a mixed fruit salad with strawberries.

FULL NAME: José Carlos Altuve

HEIGHT/WEIGHT: 5'6", 165 lbs

BORN: May 6, 1990, in Puerto Cabello, Venezuela

POSITION: Second baseman

SIGNED: As an undrafted free agent in 2007

AWARDS AND RECOGNITION: 2017 World Series Champion; 6x AL All-Star; 2015 AL Gold Glove Award; 5x AL Silver Slugger Award; 3x AL batting title; 2x AL stolen base leader; 2017 AL MVP; 2017 AL Hank Aaron Award

In my refrigerator you'll always find fruit and yogurt. For a midmorning snack, I will eat yogurt and granola. Then later in the day I eat a protein bar or a smoothie for energy—especially on really active days when I need to keep my calories high. My favorite smoothie has a mix of vegetables and fruit. I like spinach with a banana and unflavored protein powder. I just add water, mix, and drink.

My biggest meal is lunch and it's usually two pieces of grilled chicken breast, a cup or half a cup of brown rice, and vegetables. I also eat big salads with lettuce, tomatoes, and all kinds of vegetables. And then for dinner, I usually have more protein and vegetables, but fewer carbohydrates than at breakfast or lunch. I find that eating this way works best for my body and helps my performance on the field. I feel strong and energized. But I also know that I need to maintain a certain level of body fat and not get too lean because it can affect my power. I know when I'm hitting well and I know when I'm not, and sometimes it is as simple as needing to balance my intake of carbohydrates.

> *"Once I started eating better, I noticed a 100 percent change. Now I can play all season and I still feel great after it's over. After the season, I still want to go out there and play baseball. I feel faster, and after a game I sleep better. I feel very healthy."*

I recently discovered that I like fish, and will usually choose salmon or sea bass. Yesterday I had red snapper. I put it in the oven with just a little olive oil. But once a week I just eat whatever I feel like eating. A once-a-week treat is good for my mind and my body.

I got some great wellness advice from my teammate Carlos Correa. He showed up to training camp one year in really good physical shape. At the time, I was trying to get to the same place because I wanted to become a better player. So Carlos gave me some great advice: "You have to eat well. If you eat well, you're going to look good and feel good, and you're going to go out there and play well." Even though it seems like obvious advice, I always remembered it.

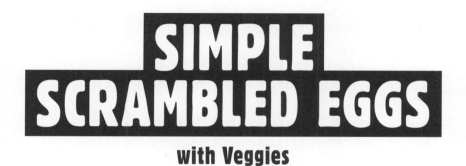

SIMPLE SCRAMBLED EGGS

with Veggies

SERVES: *1* // **PREP:** *15 minutes* // **COOK:** *5 minutes*

This is a no-fuss alternative to José Altuve's everyday omelet that is reminiscent of his Venezuelan roots. The added vegetables give these eggs a delicious and healthy boost.

2 large eggs

1½ teaspoons coconut oil

1 tablespoon finely diced onion

½ teaspoon minced garlic

½ cup chopped tomatoes

2 cups chopped baby spinach

Salt and freshly ground pepper

1. In a small bowl, whisk the eggs. Set aside.

2. In a small skillet, heat the oil over medium-high heat and cook the onion and garlic, stirring frequently, until softened, about 2 minutes. Add the tomatoes and cook, stirring frequently, for about 30 seconds.

3. Pour in the eggs and continue to stir the mixture with a rubber spatula until the eggs begin to scramble, about 1 minute. Turn off the heat and add the spinach. Cover to allow the spinach to wilt, about 30 seconds. Fold in the spinach and season with salt and pepper to taste.

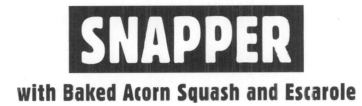

SNAPPER

with Baked Acorn Squash and Escarole

SERVES: *2* // **PREP:** *20 minutes* // **COOK:** *1 hour 10 minutes*

José Altuve knows a thing or two about big hits on the field—now here is one off the field! The roasted spiced acorn squash is what makes this entire recipe. Sometimes snapper is hard to find; striped bass works really well too.

2 snapper or striped bass fillets (4 ounces each), with skin

1 small (about 1¼ pounds) acorn squash, halved and seeds removed

3 teaspoons coconut oil, melted

4 small garlic cloves, smashed

¼ teaspoon ground cumin

¼ teaspoon cayenne

Salt and freshly ground pepper

4 small shallots, peeled and quartered

4 cups chopped escarole or watercress

1. Preheat the oven to 400°F.

2. Holding a sharp knife at a 45-degree angle, score just the skin of the snapper, making a crosshatch pattern to prevent curling while cooking. Set aside.

3. Rub the flesh side of the acorn squash with 1 teaspoon of the oil and place both halves on a large baking sheet, cut-side up. Bake for 30 minutes. Place 2 of the garlic cloves in each squash half and season with the cumin, cayenne, and salt and pepper to taste. Continue baking for 30 to 40 minutes, until the squash and the garlic are fork tender and can be easily mashed.

4. While the squash is still baking, toss the shallots in a small bowl with salt and pepper and ½ teaspoon of the coconut oil. Lay the shallots cut-side down on the baking sheet and bake for about 20 minutes, until carmelized. Reserve the shallots.

5. Scoop the flesh from the squash into a large bowl, discarding the skin, and mash it with the garlic until almost smooth. Season with salt and pepper to taste and cover to keep warm.

6. In a nonstick medium skillet, heat the remaining 1½ teaspoons oil over medium-high heat, until hot but not smoking. Place the fish in the pan skin-side down. Using an offset spatula to hold the fish flat for a few minutes to further prevent curling, cook for 3 to 4 minutes, until the skin is golden brown. Flip the fish and continue to cook about 2 minutes more, until the fish is just cooked through.

7. Transfer the fish to a plate and cover to keep warm. Add the escarole to the same skillet with a couple drops of water and cook, stirring, for about 30 seconds, until just wilted. Remove from the heat and stir in the reserved shallots. Season with salt and pepper to taste. Serve the fish with the squash and escarole alongside.

COCONUT MANGO BARS

SERVES: *12* // **PREP:** *10 minutes*

The chewy goodness of all-natural sweetness in every bite is why you won't be able to eat just one bar. Make a big batch and refrigerate in an airtight container for up to three months so you can enjoy them to your heart's content.

1 cup raw cashews
½ cup raw whole almonds
1 cup pitted dates
1 cup chopped dried apricots
½ cup chopped dried mango
½ cup unsweetened shredded coconut

1. In a food processor, blend all ingredients for 2 to 3 minutes, until well combined and sticky. On a baking sheet, shape the mixture into a rectangle 8½ x 4 x ¾ inches and refrigerate, covered, for at least 1 hour.

2. Cut into 12 bars. The bars will keep in the refrigerator, wrapped in wax paper in a sealed plastic bag or airtight container, for about 3 months.

▲ CINNAMON ALMOND
FIG BARS

*PAGE 210
(GIANCARLO STANTON)*

▲ COCONUT
MANGO BARS

GRANOLA BITES

SERVES: *8 (2 per serving)* // **PREP:** *5 minutes* // **COOK:** *20 minutes*

Granola is a go-to topping for coconut yogurt or gluten-free oatmeal, but it also makes for a great snack on its own. These super-tasty granola bars are the perfect pick-me-ups for any time of day. Keep a jarful on hand for a quick snack. Rotating the pan halfway through the baking time is key to achieving a crunchy texture.

⅓ **cup rolled oats**

⅓ **cup unsweetened coconut flakes**

2 **tablespoons sunflower seeds**

2 **tablespoons pumpkin seeds**

2 **tablespoons sesame seeds**

2 **tablespoons mini dark chocolate chips**

3 **tablespoons almond butter**

3 **tablespoons honey**

1. Preheat the oven to 350°F.

2. In a medium bowl, combine the oats, coconut, seeds, and chocolate chips. In a medium saucepan over medium heat, melt the almond butter and honey. Remove from the heat and fold the dry ingredients into the wet.

3. Scrape the mixture onto a sheet pan lined with a nonstick silicone mat. Using a rubber spatula, shape into a 5-inch square.

4. Bake for 16 to 20 minutes, rotating the pan halfway through baking, until golden brown. Let cool before cutting into 16 pieces. Granola bites will keep in an airtight container in the refrigerator for up to 6 weeks.

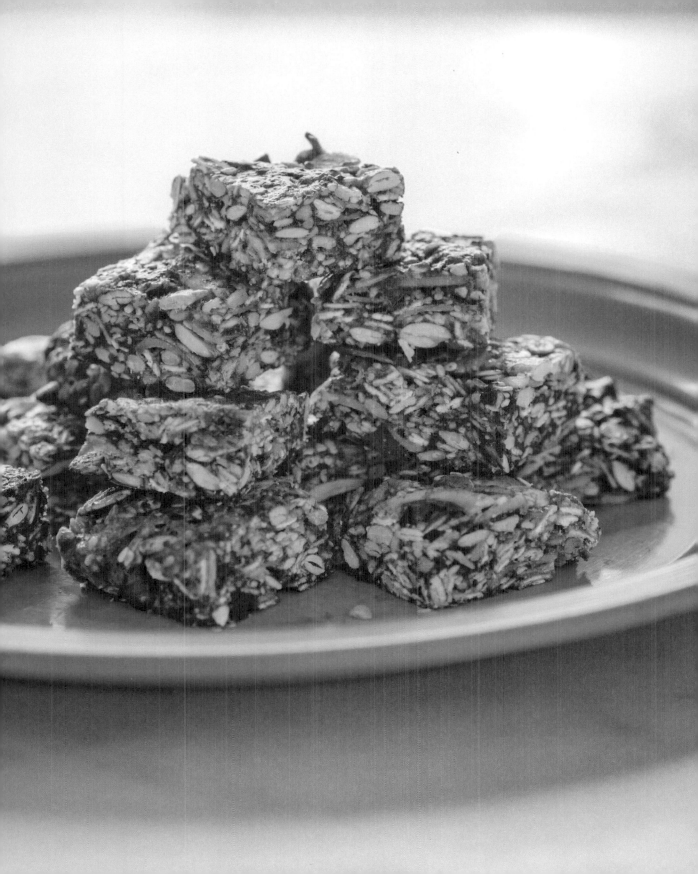

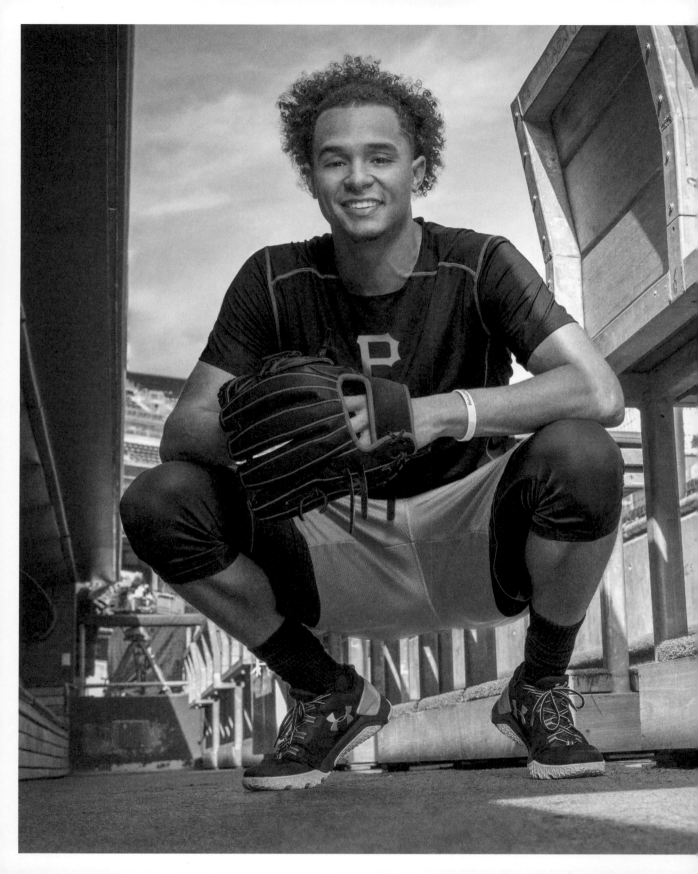

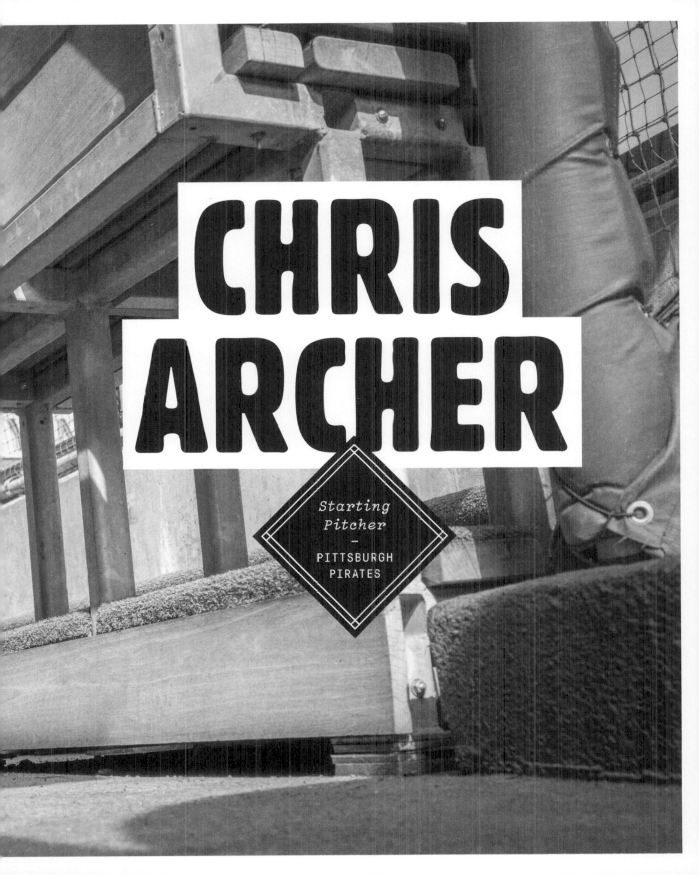

CHRIS ARCHER

Starting
Pitcher
—
PITTSBURGH
PIRATES

The person who motivated me to eat smart was my assistant football coach when I was a senior in high school. He was a former NFL player and knew more about healthy eating than anyone I have ever met. At the time, fast food was a big part of my diet. So when my coach noticed my car parked every day at a fast-food restaurant, he decided to teach me how to eat like a professional athlete. Back then I didn't have any money, and my small-town grocery store didn't have organic products, but my coach planted the seed in my mind. Two years later, I started researching nutrition and began to think of ways I could maximize my abilities and distinguish myself from other athletes with similar talent and potential. I began to look at the connections between proper sleep, working out, and nutrition.

I sleep between eight and ten hours a night. My goal is ten, but I'll never sleep less than eight hours. Our schedules are demanding, but there's always enough time to get adequate sleep. Working out without allowing yourself to get enough sleep and without putting the proper nutrients back in your body is counterproductive because your body needs to recover from exercise. I think proper nutrition and quality of sleep are often overlooked.

FULL NAME: Christopher Alan Archer

HEIGHT/WEIGHT: 6'2", 195 lbs

BORN: September 26, 1988, in Raleigh, NC

POSITION: Pitcher

DRAFT: Drafted by the Cleveland Indians in the 5th round of the 2006 MLB Draft

HIGH SCHOOL: Clayton High School (Clayton, NC)

AWARDS AND RECOGNITION: 2x AL All-Star; 2x AL most starts; on-air talent for ESPN's *Baseball Tonight*

When it comes to nutrition I'm conscious of what I put in my body, but I'm not perfect by any means. I still like pizza and chicken wings, but I'm very selective. I like to read and educate myself on a variety of ways to keep me healthy, including how proper nutrition can help prevent illness and reduce the need for taking a lot of medications.

My breakfast this morning consisted of three scrambled organic free-range eggs. But if I'm on the road, I always get poached eggs. It's the healthier way to eat eggs when you don't cook them yourself, and you don't know how they're being prepared. I also had some of yesterday's leftover green beans because I needed some greens, along with a handful of blueberries and raspberries. Usually, I have a carbohydrate in the morning, but I knew I was going to be eating carbs for lunch in four hours, and I didn't want to overload on them.

For lunch today, I had a six-ounce grilled salmon fillet with a brown rice and quinoa blend and sautéed kale. I have a variation of the same breakfast and lunch every day. And I always try to eat wild fish, organic produce, organic free-range chicken, and grass-fed meat. I try to avoid dairy and gluten because they can cause inflammation in the body.

During games, I always have a bag of mixed organic nuts and berries on hand for an energy boost. The nuts have good fats you can burn off quickly after a lot of intense physical activity. And when I need help speeding muscle recovery after a tough workout I'll just eat a handful of berries—I love blackberries, blueberries, and raspberries.

My favorite green vegetables are spinach, broccoli, kale, Brussels sprouts, asparagus, and zucchini. I go through phases, though. I prefer eating my vegetables steamed and plain with maybe a little bit of Himalayan salt, but no butter. I know grass-fed butter and ghee are considered healthy right now, but I don't like the taste of butter at all.

My favorite smoothie is one with almond butter and half a banana. Usually, I don't eat dairy because it is inflammatory, but occasionally I add in a little Greek yogurt for extra calories when I have a hard time maintaining weight. I'll also add a vegetable protein, so I am not consuming so much dairy or animal product.

When I am on the road with the team I find a health food store and get some basic things to eat like fish, chicken, quinoa, and kale salads. I always try to make the best possible choices since I can't prepare anything myself. You'll always find water, almond milk, fruit, maybe some guacamole, and nuts in my refrigerator at home.

Eating smart is definitely a process of changing your palate, especially when you're used to the richness of certain foods. I've started adding coconut oil to a lot of meals and snacks. A decent snack for me is almond butter and coconut oil on gluten-free bread. It's a healthy treat, but you have good fats, and you have a more sustainable carbohydrate.

Playing professional baseball motivates me to eat well, but the main reason I'm so conscious of nutrition is for long-term quality of life. I just try to make the best possible choices I can about eating well. I want to delay taking any medications for as long as I can. If I live eighty years, I want to live eighty quality years.

The same way we feed our bodies, we should be feeding our minds, which is why I always try to read and educate myself. I'm extremely spiritual in the sense that I believe everything is happening *for* you, not *to* you or *against* you. You just have to open your eyes and recognize that the world is not out to get you. It's especially important to remember that during tough moments. I try to learn from every situation and understand what the universe is trying to teach me about myself so I can become the best human being possible.

POACHED EGGS
with Kale and Avocado Pesto

SERVES: *2* // **PREP:** *10 minutes* // **COOK:** *10 minutes*

This easy kale and avocado pesto is enhanced with nutty, cheesy nutritional yeast and is a great accompaniment to simple poached eggs. Nutritional yeast is loaded with protein and vitamin B-12, and can be sprinkled on almost anything—making it the ideal ingredient when cheese cravings strike nondairy eaters like Chris Archer.

1 teaspoon pumpkin seeds, toasted

2 cups chopped curly kale leaves, tough ribs removed first

1 ripe avocado, cut into chunks

2 tablespoons extra-virgin olive oil

1 tablespoon fresh lime juice

1½ teaspoons nutritional yeast

1 garlic clove, grated

Pinch of crushed red pepper flakes

Salt and freshly ground pepper

Poached Eggs (recipe follows)

1. Preheat the oven to 375°F.

2. Spread the pumpkin seeds on a baking sheet and toast for 6 minutes, until they just begin to brown. Set aside.

3. In a food processor, pulse the kale, avocado, oil, lime juice, nutritional yeast, garlic, and red pepper flakes until somewhat smooth but still textured, about 30 pulses. Season with salt and pepper to taste.

4. Divide the pesto between 2 plates. Place 2 eggs on top of the pesto in each plate and sprinkle with toasted pumpkin seeds.

POACHED EGGS

2 tablespoons distilled white vinegar

4 large eggs

1. In a medium saucepan, bring 4 cups water to a slow simmer over medium heat. Add the vinegar.

2. Crack 1 egg into a small bowl, then gently slide it into the water. Repeat with the remaining eggs. Be sure the water continues to slowly bubble as the eggs set and become solid enough to remove with a slotted spoon. Poach the eggs for 3 to 4 minutes for a runny yolk and 6 to 7 minutes for a harder one.

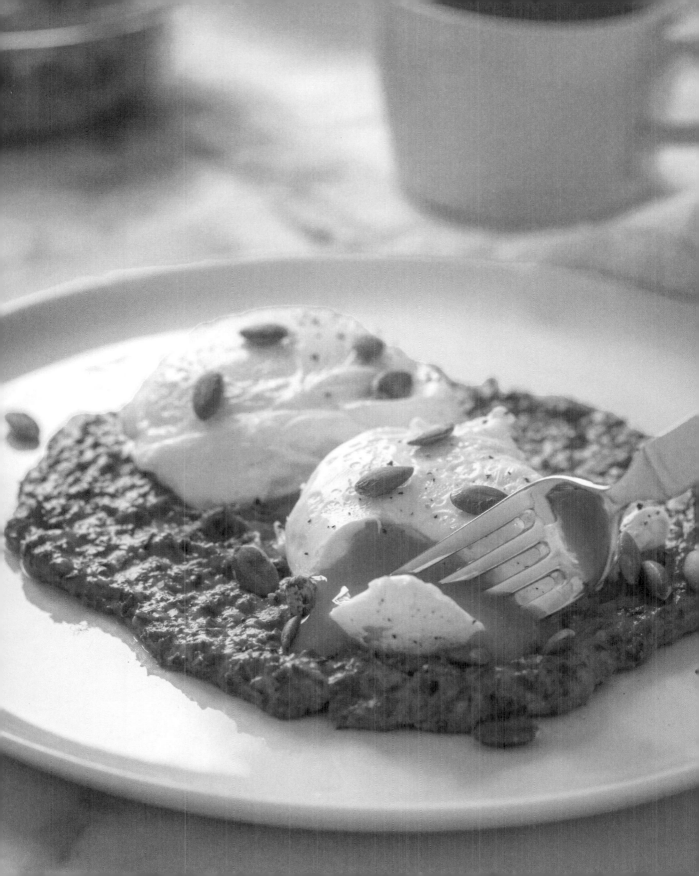

GREEN RICE BOWL

SERVES: *2* // **PREP:** *20 minutes* // **COOK:** *20 minutes*

Light and flavorful, this nourishing and versatile meal is not limited to lunch or dinner. Quick to put together, it can also be a side dish or topped with eggs for a hearty breakfast.

2 tablespoons pumpkin seeds

1½ teaspoons coconut oil, melted

1 cup quartered and trimmed Brussels sprouts

½ cup thinly sliced fennel

½ cup peeled, trimmed, and quartered pearl onions

Salt and freshly ground pepper to taste

2 cups small broccoli florets

2 tablespoons extra-virgin olive oil

2½ tablespoons fresh lime juice

1½ teaspoons grated lime zest

½ teaspoon finely grated peeled ginger root

2 cups cooked short-grain brown rice (see page 13)

2 cups chopped dinosaur kale, tough ribs removed first

1. Preheat the oven to 375°F.

2. Spread the pumpkin seeds on a baking sheet and toast for 6 minutes until they just begin to brown. Set aside.

3. Raise the oven temperature to 425°F.

4. On a baking sheet, toss the coconut oil, Brussels sprouts, fennel, and onions with salt and pepper to taste. Roast in the middle of the oven for 12 to 15 minutes, stirring halfway, until tender.

5. Meanwhile, in a saucepan fitted with a steamer basket, bring 1 inch of water to a boil. Add the broccoli, cover, and steam for 1 to 1½ minutes, until tender. Remove from the basket and set aside.

6. In a large bowl, whisk together the olive oil, lime juice and zest, and ginger. Add the roasted vegetables and broccoli and toss to combine. Season with salt and pepper to taste.

7. In a saucepan fitted with a steamer basket, bring 1 inch of water to a boil. Add the kale, cover, and steam for 1 minute. Remove from the basket.

8. Stir the rice and kale into the dressed vegetables until well combined. Divide between 2 serving bowls. Serve topped with the toasted pumpkin seeds.

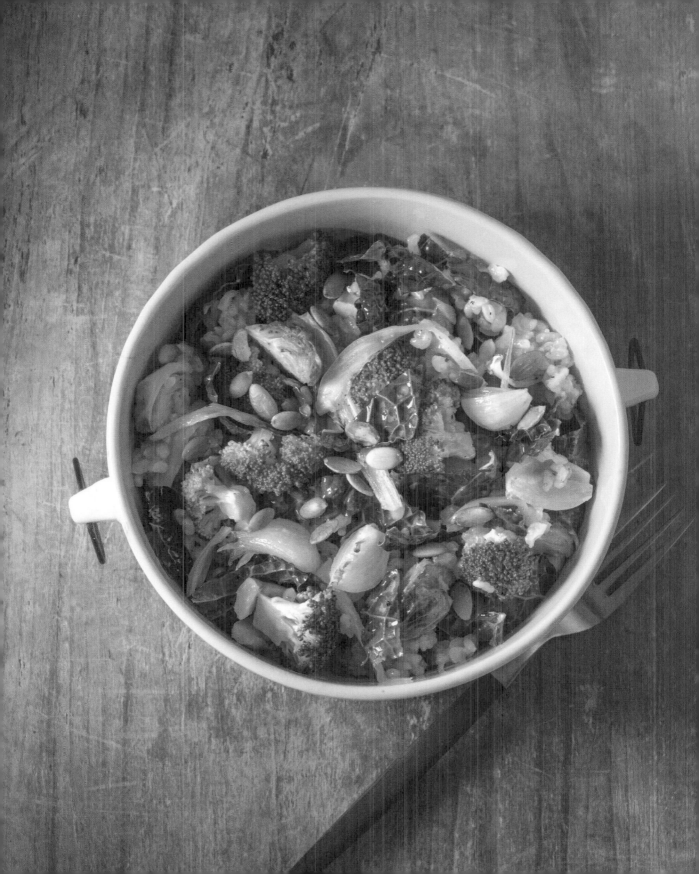

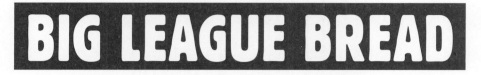

BIG LEAGUE BREAD

SERVES: *6* // **PREP:** *15 minutes* // **COOK:** *45 minutes*

Coconut nectar is a low-glycemic natural sweetener and an excellent alternative to the sugary sweeteners found in many store-bought breads. Most grocery stores stock it next to other natural sweeteners like maple syrup and honey. To keep this gluten-free bread fresh and delicious for up to 10 days, wrap it tightly and store it in the refrigerator.

2 tablespoons coconut oil, melted, plus 2 teaspoons to grease the baking dish

¾ cup oat flour, plus 2 teaspoons to dust the baking dish

1½ cups almond flour

¾ cup garbanzo flour

2 teaspoons baking soda

¾ teaspoon salt

5 large eggs

½ cup unsweetened almond milk

2 tablespoons coconut nectar

1 teaspoon cider vinegar

2 tablespoons pumpkin or sunflower seeds (optional)

1. Preheat the oven to 350°F.

2. Coat a glass 5 x 9-inch loaf pan with the 2 teaspoons oil and an even dusting of oat flour. In a large bowl, combine the almond flour, ¾ cup oat flour, garbanzo flour, baking soda, and salt. In a medium bowl, whisk together the eggs, milk, nectar, vinegar, and 2 tablespoons coconut oil. Add this mixture to the dry ingredients and mix thoroughly.

3. Pour into the loaf pan, smoothing the top, and sprinkle evenly with seeds, if using. Bake for 45 to 50 minutes, until a toothpick inserted in the center comes out clean. Allow the bread to fully cool before slicing. Covered tightly in plastic wrap and refrigerated, the bread will keep for up to 1½ weeks.

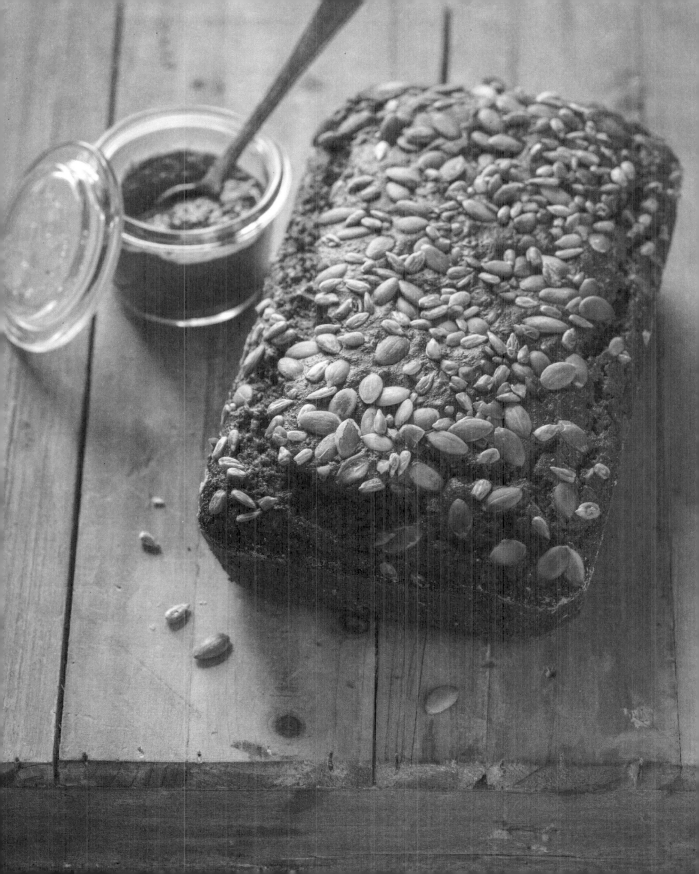

TWO-SEAMER TOAST

with Almond Butter and Blackberry Jam

SERVES: *1* // MAKES: *2 toasts with 2 tablespoons almond butter and 2 tablespoons jam* // PREP: *5 minutes*

This clean take on a traditional PB&J is mouthwateringly good. Coconut sugar in place of granulated sugar is the healthier way to go when making jam. Blackberries are a great fruit for making jam and a favorite of Chris Archer's, but almost any kind of berries can be used to make this childhood treat.

2 (½-inch-thick) slices of gluten-free bread (such as **Big League Bread, page 34**), toasted

2 tablespoons almond butter

2 tablespoons Blackberry Jam (recipe follows)

Toast the bread until golden. Spread 1 tablespoon almond butter on each slice. Spoon 1 tablespoon blackberry jam over each piece of toast and spread to cover.

BLACKBERRY JAM

SERVES: *1* // PREP: *5 minutes* // COOK: *25 minutes*

1 pint blackberries, halved

1 tablespoon coconut sugar

In a medium saucepan, bring the blackberries, sugar, and 1 cup water to a simmer over medium-low heat. Simmer, stirring occasionally, until the fruit reaches a jamlike consistency, about 25 minutes. Let the jam cool before refrigerating in an airtight container. The jam will keep for up to 2 months.

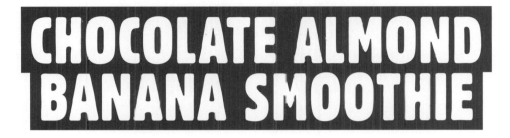

CHOCOLATE ALMOND BANANA SMOOTHIE

SERVES: *1* // **PREP:** *5 minutes*

Maintaining weight for some athletes, including Chris Archer, is sometimes challenging. This rich smoothie is full of healthy fats without any added dairy or refined sugar. For the banana, frozen is best for providing a hint of coolness without adding ice.

1½ cups chilled coconut milk (see page 13)
1 tablespoon almond butter
1 ripe banana, sliced (frozen is best)
1½ teaspoons unsweetened cacao powder
1 tablespoon hemp hearts
1½ teaspoons cacao nibs (optional)
3 mint leaves (optional)
Pinch of cayenne (optional)

In a high-powered blender, combine the milk, almond butter, banana, cacao powder, and hemp hearts (and the cacao nibs, mint, and/or cayenne, if using) and process until smooth.

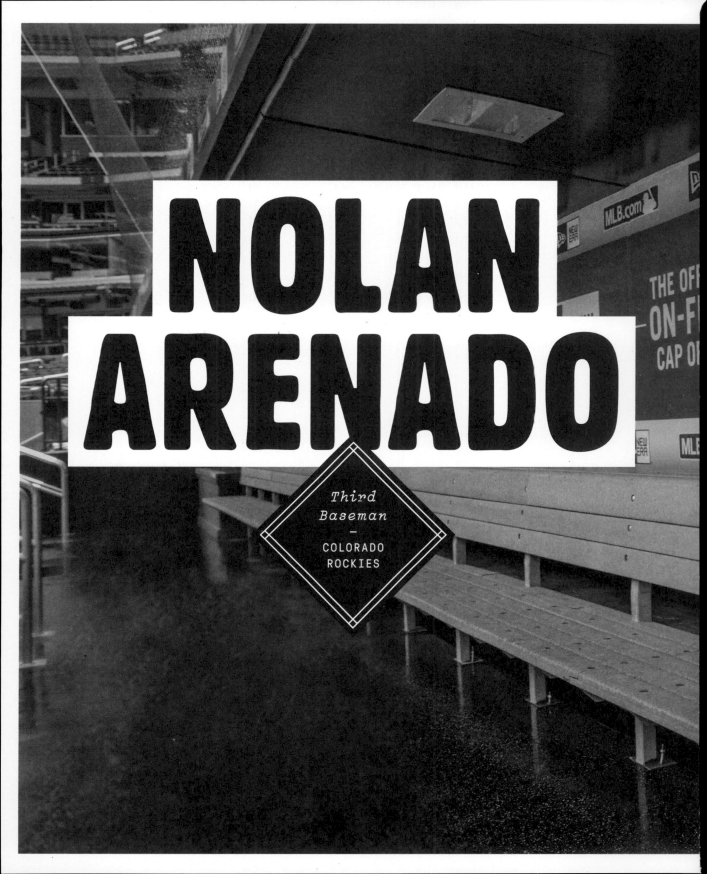

NOLAN ARENADO

Third Baseman
—
COLORADO
ROCKIES

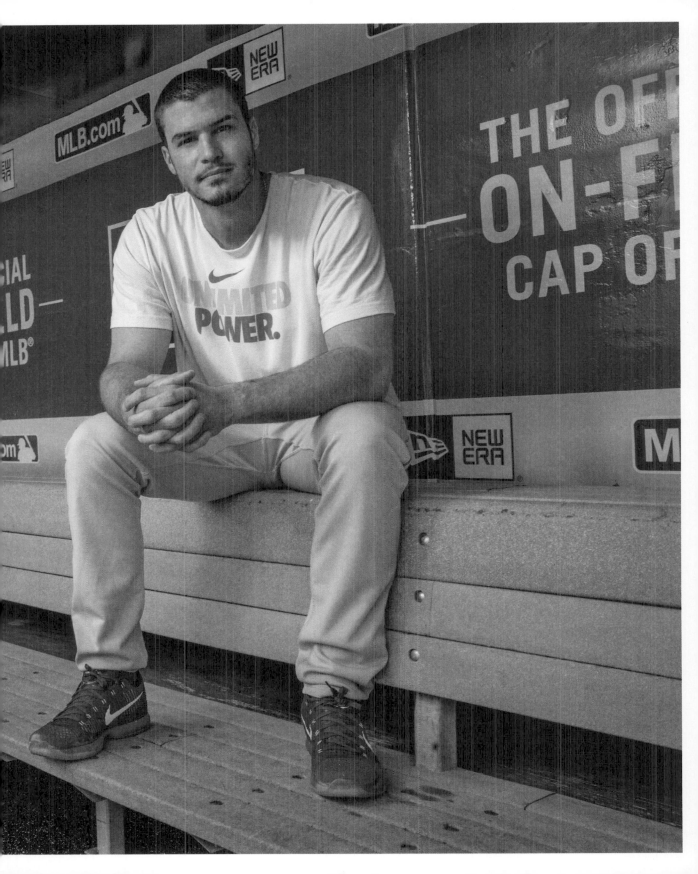

My motivation to eat well started when I was in the Minor Leagues. I weighed 240 pounds at my first Spring Training. I felt terrible. I was weak and slow. In the off-season, I got a nutritionist and changed my eating habits so I wouldn't end up in fat camp during the next Spring Training.

One of the biggest changes I made to my diet was fixing the bad eating habits I developed growing up. I'm Cuban and I love Cuban food, which we all know can be delicious but also fattening. The first two weeks of changing my diet were tough, but after that I started feeling better and locked in to my new way of eating. And once you're in that zone, the unhealthy food you once craved doesn't taste good anymore and makes your body feel terrible.

By cutting back on sugar and any form of bread at night my weight got down to 210. If I did eat sugar I wouldn't have it later than six at night because there's no time to burn it off before bed. It's harder to lose the weight when you eat sugary foods late in the day because your body is inactive and not burning calories. Also, I switched from coffee to tea. I transformed everything about my diet.

FULL NAME: Nolan James Arenado

HEIGHT/WEIGHT: 6'2", 205 lbs

BORN: April 16, 1991, in Newport Beach, CA

POSITION: Third baseman

DRAFT: Drafted by the Colorado Rockies in the 2nd round of the 2009 MLB Draft

HIGH SCHOOL: El Toro High School (Lake Forest, CA)

AWARDS AND RECOGNITION: 4x NL All-Star; 6x NL Gold Glove Award; 4x NL Silver Slugger Award; 2x NL home run leader; 2x NL RBI leader; hit for cycle on June 18, 2017

I have a lot more energy and am performing better on the field now that I eat well. When I was in the Minors I would sleep until one o'clock in the afternoon and then grab fast food. Now I wake up at ten in the morning and have a well-balanced breakfast. I'm more energized and ready to go to the ballpark.

On game days I eat oatmeal with fruit for breakfast—it feels light and I can use those carbs throughout the day until game time. I also drink two full bottles of water in the morning. The Denver altitude can be tough so it's important to always stay hydrated, especially for recovery. I always make sure I replenish throughout the day and eat enough.

In my refrigerator, you'll always find turkey burger patties ready to go so that I have something to cook in a pinch. I usually have strawberries and all sorts of vegetables on hand too. I really love bell peppers. I never liked broccoli, but now I'm okay with it, and mushrooms too. I love Brussels sprouts. They're my new favorite. I'm all about these vegetables now—they're actually good!

> *"When you work out and eat right, your confidence goes through the roof. And when you're confident, you play better."*

I try to stay away from eating processed carbohydrates, so it's rare that I will eat bread. I'll have cheat meals once in a while, but I usually stick with the same foods: After a tough workout, my go-to is steak with brown rice and black beans. Lunch is usually a mixed bowl of brown rice, black beans, chicken, and vegetables. It can be a different mix of foods so long as I eat a balance of protein and carbs. It's not heavy and I feel light and not achy. And for dinner after a game I'll have something similar, but I might have fish or steak instead of chicken. I like all white fish, especially halibut, and I like asparagus. After every game, I also drink chocolate milk because it is supposed to help with muscle recovery.

My former teammate Troy Tulowitzki emphasized the importance of being lean, which was a great piece of advice. Being lean makes me more agile, quicker, and explosive on the field. It has affected my performance. Once I started leaning out, I noticed a difference in my play. I never want to be the baseball player who's overweight. I want to make sure I'm coming into the season ready to go. I can feel it in my body. When you work out and eat right, your confidence goes through the roof. And when you're confident, you play better.

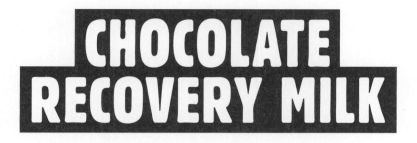

CHOCOLATE RECOVERY MILK

SERVES: *4* // **PREP:** *5 minutes*

Nolan Arenado's favored chocolate milk for muscle recovery gets a reboot minus the dairy. Raw honey replaces the refined sugars found in store-bought chocolate milk, and coconut water adds essential electrolytes. It's a game-ending walk-off hit.

1½ cups chilled unsweetened almond milk (see page 13)

1½ cups chilled coconut water

1 ripe banana

2 tablespoons unsweetened cacao powder

1 tablespoon raw honey

Half a vanilla bean, split and seeds scraped (you should have about ½ teaspoon seeds)

In a high-powered blender, combine the almond milk, coconut water, banana, cacao powder, honey, and vanilla seeds and process until smooth.

CUBAN BLACK BEANS
with Jicama Rice

SERVES: *2* // **PREP:** *25 minutes* // **COOK:** *10 minutes*

The sweet and refreshing tastes of kohlrabi and jicama add a delicious complexity to a familiar Cuban staple that is a favorite of Nolan Arenado's. As a meal or side dish, it's so good you'll want to double the recipe.

1½ cups diced peeled jicama

1 cup diced bell peppers

½ cup diced peeled kohlrabi

3 tablespoons finely diced red onion

1 tablespoon fresh lime juice

Salt and freshly ground pepper

1½ cups sugar snap peas

2 teaspoons coconut oil

3 tablespoons finely diced yellow onion

1 teaspoon minced garlic

2 cups cooked black beans (see page 12) with 1 cup cooking liquid

½ teaspoon dried oregano

¼ teaspoon ground cumin

½ ripe avocado, sliced

1. Place the jicama in a food processor. Pulse about 20 times, stopping midway through to scrape down the sides, until it looks like rice. Place the jicama in a bowl with the peppers, kohlrabi, red onion, and lime juice. Toss to combine with salt and pepper to taste.

2. In a saucepan fitted with a steamer basket, bring 1 inch of water to a boil. Put the snap peas in the basket, cover, and steam for 1 minute. Remove from the basket and set aside.

3. Heat the oil in a medium saucepan. Add the yellow onion and garlic and cook, stirring, until golden, about 2 minutes. Stir in the beans with their liquid, oregano, and cumin. Simmer for 8 to 10 minutes, until the liquid is reduced and coats the beans. Remove from the heat and season with salt and pepper to taste.

4. Divide the jicama-rice mixture between 2 bowls. Spoon black beans, snap peas, and avocado around it.

HALIBUT

with Spiced Sweet Potato Mash and Roasted Asparagus

SERVES: 2 // **PREP:** 15 minutes // **COOK:** 1 hour

Halibut tastes best when simply prepared, whether seared, roasted, or grilled. The subtly spiced sweet potato and roasted asparagus make this dinner a star.

1 large sweet potato

½ pound asparagus, trimmed

2 tablespoons thinly sliced Vidalia onion

3 teaspoons coconut oil

Salt and freshly ground pepper

2 teaspoons extra-virgin olive oil

½ teaspoon ground cumin

½ teaspoon ground coriander

2 (1-inch thick) halibut fillets (4 ounces each), skin removed

2 teaspoons fresh lemon juice

1. Preheat the oven to 375°F.

2. Place the sweet potato on a baking sheet and bake for 40 to 45 minutes, until soft.

3. Preheat the broiler. On a baking sheet, toss the asparagus with the onion, 1 teaspoon of the coconut oil, and salt and pepper to taste. Broil 6 inches from the heat for 6 to 8 minutes, stirring occasionally, until golden brown and tender. Set aside.

4. Remove the skin from the sweet potato. In a bowl, mash with 1 teaspoon of the olive oil, the cumin, coriander, and salt and pepper to taste.

5. Heat the remaining 2 teaspoons coconut oil in a small nonstick skillet over medium-high heat. Season the halibut with salt and pepper and place in the hot oil to begin searing. Reduce the heat to medium and continue to sear for 2½ to 3 minutes before flipping the fish. Cook the second side until cooked through and opaque, about 3 minutes more.

6. Divide the sweet potato mash and the asparagus between 2 plates, placing the asparagus alongside the potato. Set one halibut fillet on each plate.

7. Combine the lemon juice with the remaining 1 teaspoon olive oil and drizzle over the fish.

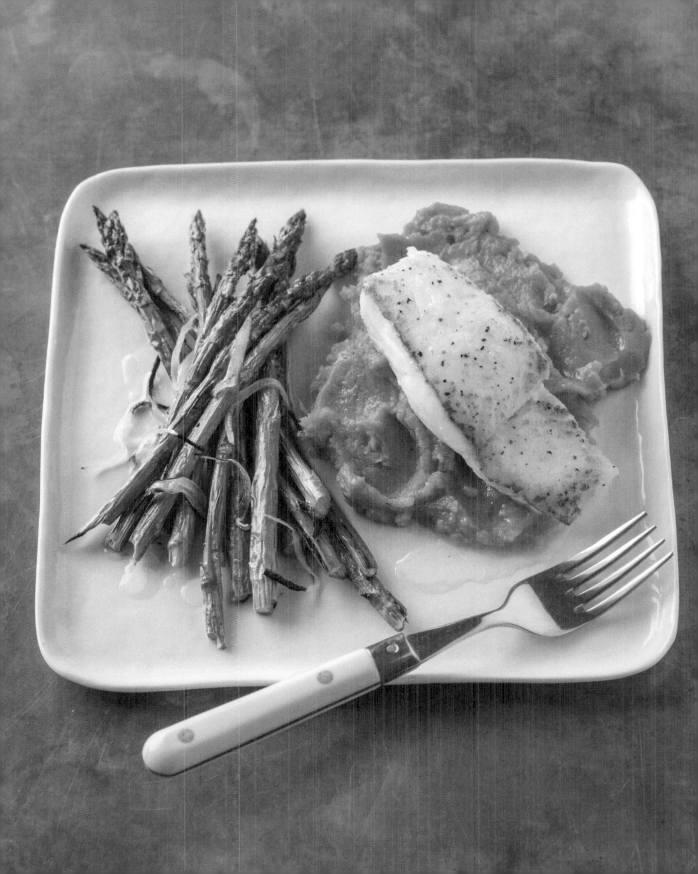

ROASTED MUSHROOM

Rice Bowl with Watercress

SERVES: *2* // **PREP:** *35 minutes* // **COOK:** *40 minutes*

Broiled sunchokes are an unexpected addition to this delectable rice bowl. Watercress, a superfood with potent nutrients, creates a peppery counterpoint to the earthy mushroom and rice flavors.

¼ ounce dried porcini

1½ cups diced peeled sunchokes

1 tablespoon plus 3½ teaspoons coconut oil, melted

Salt and freshly ground pepper

12 ounces mushrooms (shiitake, maitake, portobello, button, or a mix)

12 Brussels sprouts

2 tablespoons thinly sliced shallots

2 cups cooked short-grain brown rice (see page 13)

2 teaspoons finely chopped fresh thyme

2 handfuls of watercress

2 lemon wedges

1. In a saucepan over medium heat, bring the porcini and 2 cups water to a simmer and cook for 25 to 30 minutes, until reduced to ½ cup. Strain the broth, reserving the liquid, and dice the mushrooms. Set aside.

2. Preheat the broiler. Toss the sunchokes with 1½ teaspoons of the oil and season with salt and pepper to taste. Arrange in one layer on a baking sheet. Broil 6 inches from heat for 8 to 12 minutes, stirring occasionally, until golden brown and tender. Set aside.

3. If using portobello or button, trim bottoms of stems (remove shiitake stems completely) and slice the mushrooms into ¼-inch strips. If using maitake, break them up so they will lie flat. Place the mushrooms on a baking sheet and toss with 2 teaspoons of the oil and season with salt and pepper to taste. Broil 6 inches from the heat for 5 minutes, stirring occasionally, until golden. Remove from the oven and, when cool enough to handle, chop into bite-size pieces.

4. Using a paring knife, trim the stem end of each Brussels sprout and peel away the outer leaves. Continue trimming and peeling until all the leaves are separated. In a saucepan fitted with a steamer basket, bring 1 inch of water to a boil. Put the Brussels sprout leaves in the basket, cover, and steam for 45 seconds.

5. Heat the remaining 1 tablespoon of oil in a large saucepan over medium heat. Add the shallots and cook for 2 to 3 minutes, until they start to brown. Add the reserved mushroom broth and porcinis, sunchokes, rice, Brussels sprout leaves, and thyme. Stir until heated through, about 1 minute. Season with salt and pepper to taste.

6. Place a handful of watercress in each of 2 bowls. Divide the rice mixture between the bowls. Squeeze a lemon wedge over top.

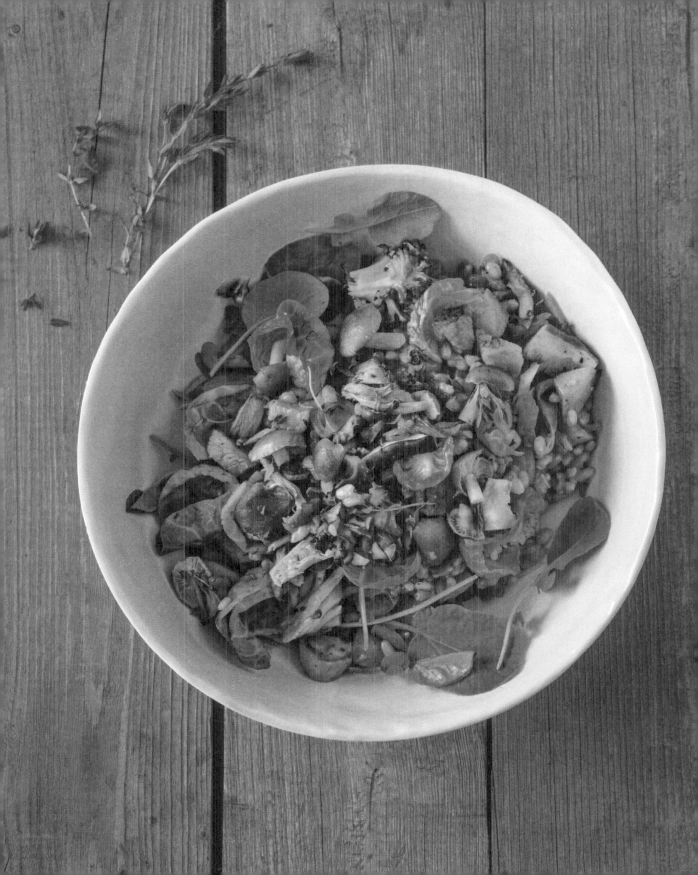

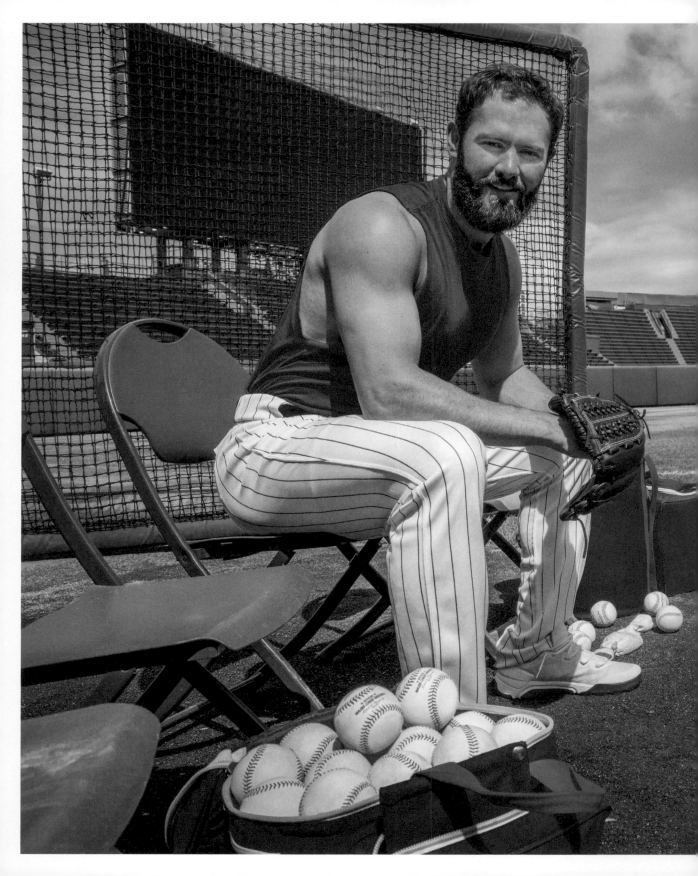

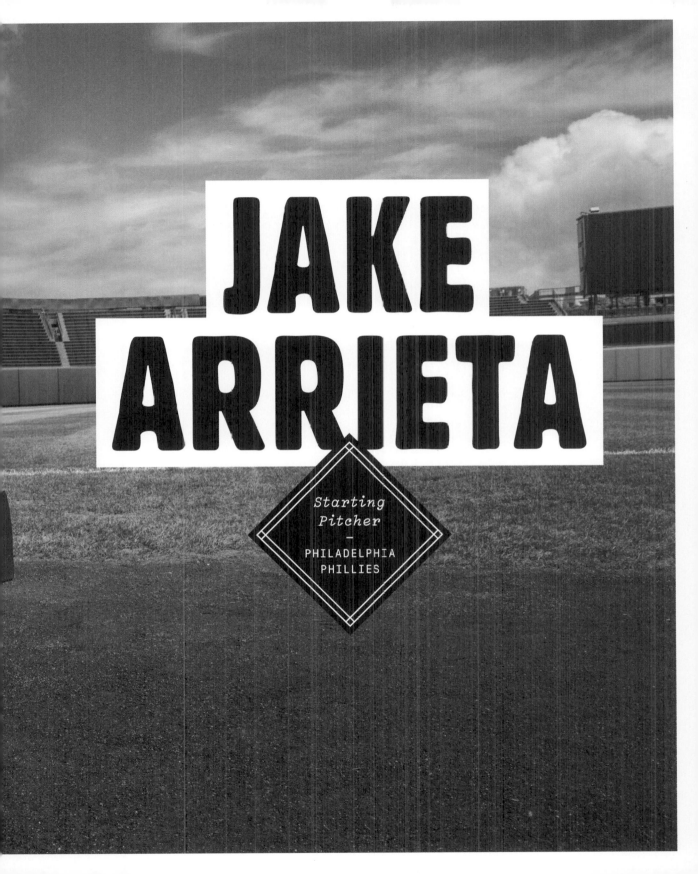

JAKE ARRIETA

Starting Pitcher
—
PHILADELPHIA PHILLIES

Eating smart is part of my job description—if I want to play this game for a long time, I have to recognize that my body is a machine and I'm going to get out of it what I put in. Once I started understanding how nutrition and sports go hand in hand, I was intrigued to learn that a healthy diet could drastically change my body and my energy levels.

On game days, I try to eat a light but nutrient-dense meal, which prevents me from running out of energy and crashing. Eating a proper diet helps me maintain my energy levels throughout the day, especially on the days I pitch.

For me, good nutrition is about finding balance. Not to say that I don't slip up and have my cheat days. You will absolutely drive yourself crazy if you don't, so for me, I choose to have the cheat day normally the day after I pitch. I let loose.

I've learned recently about the benefits of high-quality saturated fats like grass-fed butter. Grass-fed butter gives you a prolonged feeling of sustained energy so I always have that in my refrigerator. I'm always trying new things

FULL NAME: Jacob Joseph Arrieta

HEIGHT/WEIGHT: 6'4", 225 lbs

BORN: March 6, 1986, in Farmington, MO

POSITION: Pitcher

DRAFT: Drafted by the Cincinnati Reds in the 31st round of the 2004 MLB Draft; the Milwaukee Brewers in the 26th round of the 2005 MLB Draft; and the Baltimore Orioles in the 5th round of the 2007 MLB Draft

HIGH SCHOOL: Plano East High School (Plano, TX)

COLLEGE: Texas Christian University (Fort Worth, TX)

AWARDS AND RECOGNITION: 2016 World Series Champion (Cubs); 2016 NL All-Star; 2015 NL Cy Young Award; 2016 NL Silver Slugger Award (for best hitting pitcher); 2015 wins leader; 2 no-hitters (2015, 2016)

and I'm pretty adventurous when it comes to food.

My favorite fresh juice is any combination of celery, cucumber, kale, spinach, and parsley with a lemon or a lime, which provides a bit of sweetness without the sugar. People lose sight of the added sugar in juices. If you're drinking green juice or a smoothie with two or three apples in there and pineapple, that's adding a lot of sugar you don't necessarily need. So when I have a smoothie, I'll make sure to add a handful or two of spinach, kale, or another leafy green. I also add two to three tablespoons of hemp seeds and the same amount of flax and chia seeds. If I throw a fruit in, it's typically a banana. The liquid base is water with maybe an ounce or two of orange juice to add a little sweetness. The only time I'll drink something sweeter is when I need to speed up muscle recovery after a tough workout—then I'll have a juice with fresh pineapple, turmeric, ginger, and maybe something else to fight inflammation.

It's important to find a way to make your healthy food taste good. A lot

> "Eating smart is part of my job description—if I want to play this game for a long time, I have to recognize that my body is a machine and I'm going to get out of it what I put in. Once I started understanding how nutrition and sports go hand in hand, I was intrigued to learn that a healthy diet could drastically change my body and my energy levels."

of people are turned off by certain foods because they're bland or taste bad, but there are ways to make meals very tasty without a ton of added fat or sugar. I try to learn as much as I can about nutrition. For example, I recently read about the benefits of coconut oil and have started using it in my diet.

I am a fan of superfoods and matcha green tea. I'll buy vegan proteins and different supplements, including spirulina. I'll get out the blender, make a shake, and toss a little of all that in there. I notice I have more energy that is better sustained when I start my day this way.

When I'm on the road I bring my own healthier snack foods so I can avoid the minibar in the room. I request a refrigerator in my hotel room and I stop at a healthy grocery store wherever I am so I can keep some things on hand.

Lunch is usually a turkey BLT—I allow myself to have some more carbs than **at other meals.** I might have a burger made from grass-fed beef with sweet potato fries. But lunch is the only time I'll eat a sandwich or a burger. I just try to make sure whatever I am eating is high-quality food.

My ideal dinner would be based on vegan principles, but I find that having some animal protein in my diet helps me to maintain my strength and endurance throughout the season. I try not to eat a ton of red meat, but in moderation it's fine for me. And I love salmon, tuna, and any type of sushi. For complex carbs, sweet potatoes are my staple. I eat a lot of asparagus and broccoli. During the season I will usually have grilled chicken breast with a sweet potato, corn on the cob, broccoli, and Brussels sprouts.

Jim Palmer always said, "Health is wealth." He had a tremendous pitching career and looks great to this day.

QUINOA BURGER STACK

with Crispy Cayenne Sweet Potato Fries

SERVES: *2* // **PREP:** *30 minutes* // **COOK:** *20 minutes*

As a meal or even an hors d'oeuvre for a party, this recipe is a sure crowd pleaser. The slightly crispy sweet potato fries are the perfect complement—resist turning them too often while cooking to achieve the right amount of crispness.

4½ teaspoons coconut oil

½ cup finely chopped onion

¼ cup finely chopped carrot

¼ cup finely chopped celery

2 cups cooked quinoa (see page 13), cooled

2 tablespoons chopped fresh herbs, such as thyme, parsley, and rosemary

Salt and freshly ground pepper

Avocado Mash (recipe follows on page 54)

Crispy Cayenne Sweet Potato Fries (recipe follows on page 54)

1. In a small nonstick skillet, heat 1½ teaspoons of the oil over medium heat, then add the onion, carrot, and celery. Cover, to sweat the vegetables, stirring, until tender, about 4 minutes. Remove from the heat, uncover, and let cool.

2. Combine the vegetable mixture with the quinoa and herbs and season with salt and pepper to taste. Blend in a food processor for 30 seconds to 1 minute, until a paste forms. Shape into 6 (3-inch) patties (a scant ⅓ cup each).

3. In a large nonstick skillet, heat 1½ teaspoons of the oil over medium-high heat. Cook 3 burgers for 3 to 4 minutes on each side, until golden brown. Repeat with the remaining oil and remaining 3 patties. Top the cooked burgers with avocado mash into a 2-tiered stack or as a single layer. Serve with the sweet potato fries.

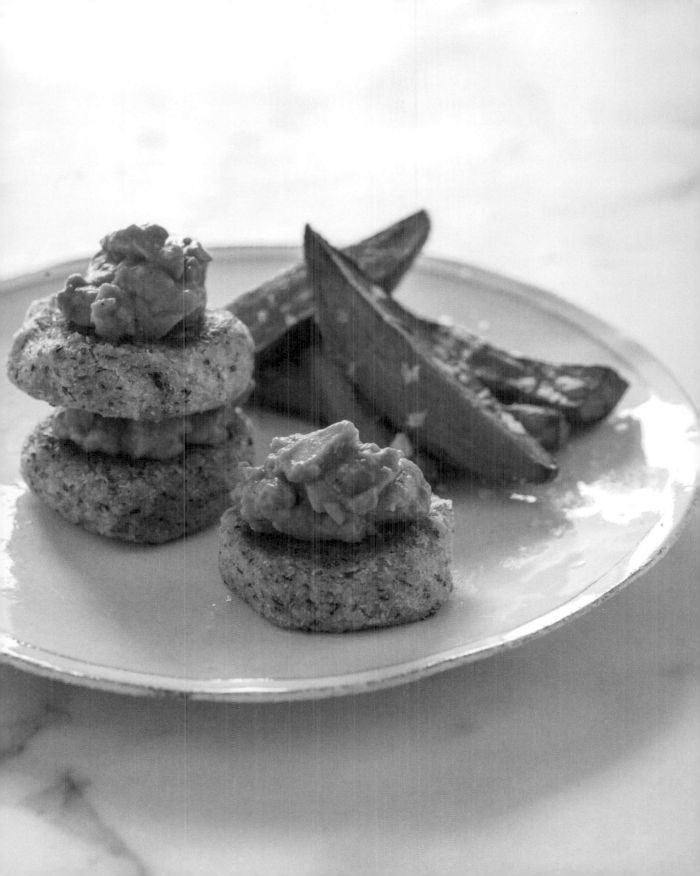

AVOCADO MASH

SERVES: 2 // **PREP:** 5 minutes

1 ripe avocado, cut into chunks

1 tablespoon fresh lime juice

1 teaspoon extra-virgin olive oil

1 tablespoon chopped fresh cilantro, or to taste (optional)

Salt and freshly ground pepper

In a small bowl, mash the avocado with the lime juice and oil. Fold in the cilantro, if using, and season with salt and pepper to taste.

CRISPY CAYENNE SWEET POTATO FRIES

SERVES: 2 // **PREP:** 5 minutes //
COOK: 1 hour

2 medium sweet potatoes, unpeeled

1½ teaspoons coconut oil, melted

⅛ teaspoon cayenne (optional)

Large flake sea salt

1. Preheat the oven to 375°F.

2. Place the sweet potatoes on a baking sheet and bake for 30 to 35 minutes, until just starting to get soft. Let cool enough to cut into wedges.

3. Toss with the oil and cayenne (if using) and season with salt to taste. Arrange the wedges cut-sides down on the baking sheet. Bake for about 30 minutes, turning halfway through, until golden brown and slightly crispy.

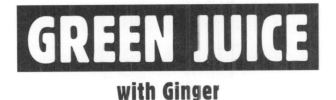

GREEN JUICE

with Ginger

SERVES: *1* // **PREP:** *10 minutes*

Resist the urge to overload fresh juice with lots of unnecessary high-glycemic fruits. Each sip of this uncomplicated green juice is clean tasting—just as Jake Arrieta likes it. The lemon and lime give it a refreshing edge and the ginger strengthens digestion.

2 cups chopped romaine

1½ cups chopped cucumber

1 cup chopped celery

1 lemon, peel removed and fruit chopped

2-inch piece of ginger root, chopped

½ lime, peel removed and fruit chopped

Pass the romaine, cucumber, celery, lemon, ginger, and lime through a juicer. When juicing, it is best not to leave the ginger until the end so that the citrus juice can help to catch any remaining ginger bits.

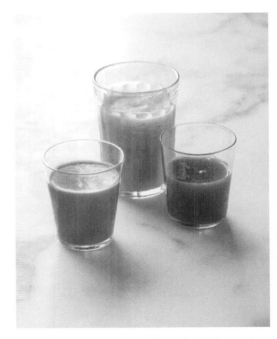

Clockwise: Green Juice; Grapefruit Turmeric Manuka Shot, page 171 *(Ian Kinsler)*; Turmeric Ginger Pineapple Shot, page 56

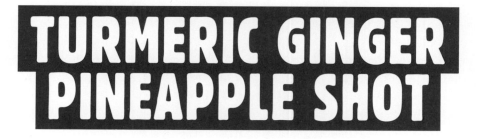

TURMERIC GINGER PINEAPPLE SHOT

SERVES: *2* // **PREP:** *10 minutes*

The ginger, turmeric, and pineapple in this shot (pictured on page 55) help ease inflammation. Be sure to wear gloves when using turmeric to avoid getting its natural amber residue on your fingertips.

1 cup chopped peeled pineapple

Two 3-inch pieces of turmeric root, chopped (about ½ cup)

2-inch piece of ginger root, chopped

Pinch of freshly ground pepper (optional)

Pass the pineapple, turmeric, and ginger through a juicer. If you like, add black pepper to increase the bioavailability of the turmeric.

MATCHA SMOOTHIE

SERVES: *1* // **PREP:** *15 minutes, plus chilling time*

Loaded with protein and an energy charge from the matcha tea, this delicious smoothie is suitable for breakfast, lunch, or any time you need a pick-me-up. Chia seeds have a tasty, nutty flavor and are rich in omega-3 fatty acids.

1 teaspoon matcha tea powder

1 small orange, peel and pith removed (discard any loose seeds) and fruit chopped

1½ cups baby spinach

1 large banana, broken into pieces

1 tablespoon flaxseeds

1 tablespoon chia seeds

1 tablespoon hemp hearts

1. In a small bowl, sift the matcha into ¾ cup warm water and whisk together until dissolved. Chill until cold.

2. In a high-powered blender, combine the chilled matcha, orange, spinach, banana, flaxseeds, chia seeds, and hemp hearts and process until smooth.

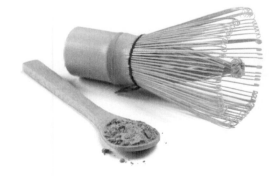

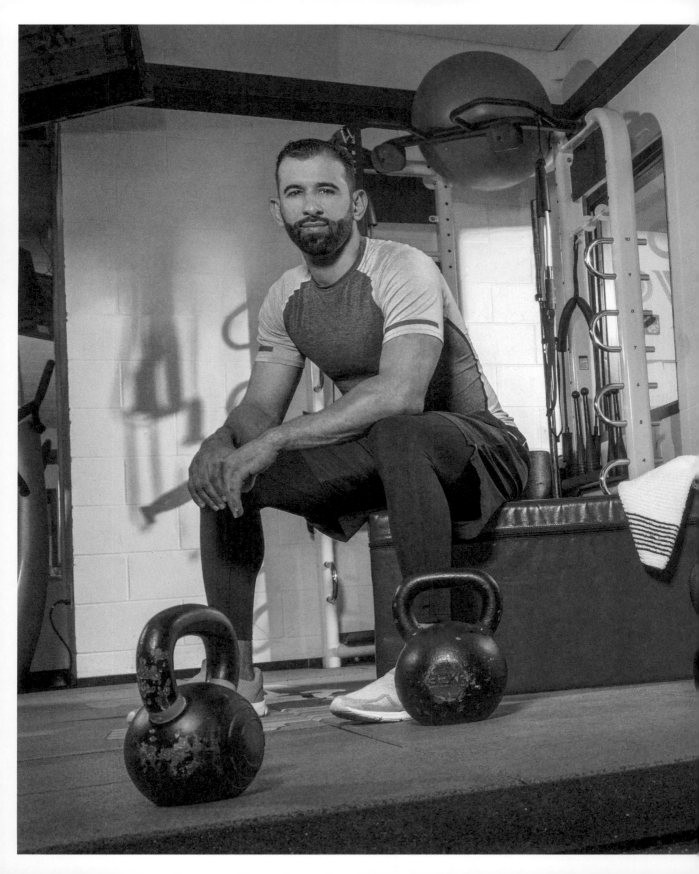

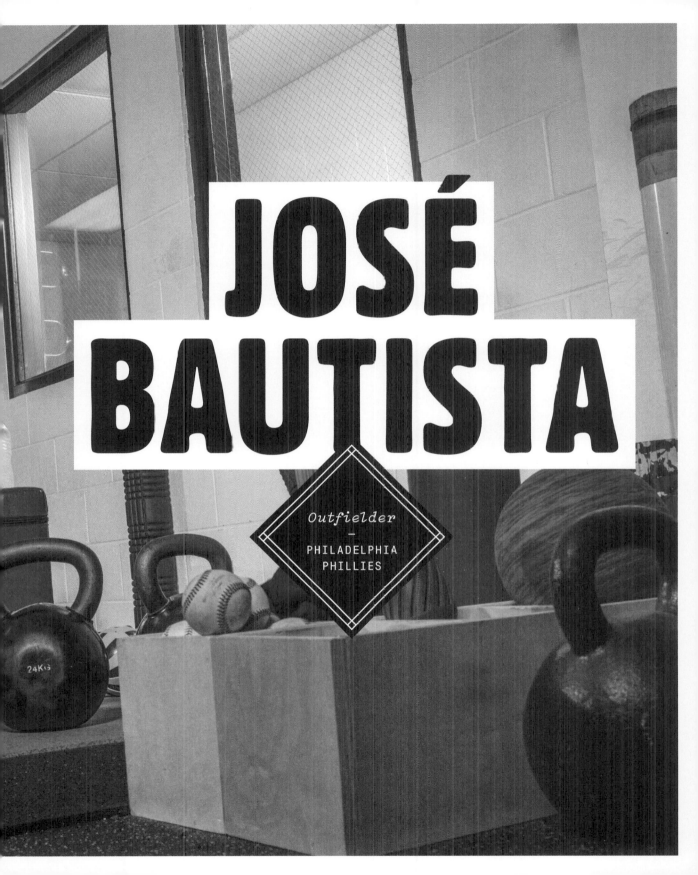

JOSÉ BAUTISTA

Outfielder
—
PHILADELPHIA PHILLIES

My body is my number one tool and I've got to take care of it. Starting in high school I was always researching the right things to eat—looking online, talking to nutritionists, dieticians, and performance experts. There have been a lot of advances over the years that have helped me narrow down what I'll eat today. Eating smart is related to what I do for a living. I deserve it, my employer deserves it, and the fans deserve it. And I'm not going to play forever, so I want to take advantage of this time in my life.

I try to add food to my diet that is going to help me heal if I'm injured or sick so that I don't have to take medicine. I pick food and seasonings that are going to be healing, not just tasty.

I have oatmeal for breakfast every day because it's not only a good gluten-free source of protein, but it also helps detox the body. I put fruit on it, along with nuts, cinnamon, nutmeg, and some cloves. I make it with almond milk.

I eliminated beef and dairy from my diet during the last off-season and I've noticed that I am less stiff and less bloated. I also have less inflammation. Cutting out sugar helps too. Sometimes

I'll have raw agave or honey, but only occasionally. When I did eat meat it was always from Colorado and grass fed.

When you're hungry and looking for a snack, reach for fruits and vegetables and you'll be fine. You'll always find fruits and vegetables in my refrigerator for that reason.

My favorite smoothie has berries in it for the antioxidants, plus almond or rice milk. I add superfoods in powder form, like protein powders with multivitamins and turmeric. I throw in Brazil nuts because they have a lot of glutathione, which is an important antioxidant that's hard to get through your diet.

I drink a lot of tea, usually with turmeric and ginger. I don't have caffeinated tea except for green tea in the morning, and even that doesn't have as much caffeine as black tea. Lately I've been on a blueberry green tea kick. After every meal, I drink some kind of tea depending on the time of day and what kind of meal I ate. If I eat a big meal I'll go with a cup of ginger mint tea. Before bed I drink chamomile. If I feel worn out after a game, I'll go for something good for recovery like coconut almond chai tea.

FULL NAME: José Antonio Bautista

HEIGHT/WEIGHT: 6'0", 205 lbs

BORN: October 19, 1980, in Santo Domingo, Dominican Republic

POSITIONS: Right fielder and third baseman

DRAFT: Drafted by the Pittsburgh Pirates in the 20th round of the 2000 MLB Draft

HIGH SCHOOL: De La Salle, Santo Domingo, Dominican Republic

AWARDS AND RECOGNITION: 6x AL All-Star; 3x AL Silver Slugger Award; 2x AL Hank Aaron Award; 2x MLB home run leader

"My favorite smoothie has berries in it for the antioxidants, plus almond or rice milk. I add superfoods in powder form, like protein powders with multivitamins and turmeric. I throw in Brazil nuts because they have a lot of glutathione, which is an important antioxidant that's hard to get through your diet."

My favorite fruits are tropical and exotic like passion fruit, mango, and papaya. They were in my diet growing up. I'm from the Dominican Republic and I'm kind of going back to my roots a little bit to bring up my immune system.

My biggest meal of the day is lunch—I normally have a gluten-free grain like rice, risotto, or quinoa with lentils, mung beans, or some other type of bean. I also have either a fish or a bird. There are always vegetables and often I add in an avocado. I like my fish or chicken sautéed with vegetables, mostly green peppers and onions. Sometimes I'll eat rice with peas in it; it's really good cooked in coconut milk. Dinner is similar to lunch but a little lighter. I throw in a salad because that helps to detox your system when you're sleeping. I like to do my detoxing at night and also when I wake up. So I'll eat salad at night and have oatmeal in the morning.

It's a cliché, but your body is your temple—you have to take care of it and know what you're putting in it. If you neglect or mistreat your body, it's going to come back to haunt you at some point. You've got to know what you're doing. Even the water you drink, which I never paid attention to before, can throw you off balance. It's so simple.

Once a week, I do a three-hour long acupuncture session and a lot of breathing exercises. This leads to a self-meditative state and helps me get rid of tension. I get massages three times a week on different days than the acupuncture. I do a lot of stress-relieving things, including cupping, to relieve tension. If tension builds up it's harder to get rid of it later. It's like ironing a shirt—if you let it get super wrinkled, you are going to have to iron it for, like, seven hours to make it flat. So if I see a little wrinkle, I take care of it right away.

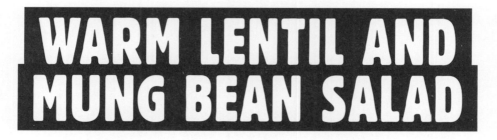

WARM LENTIL AND MUNG BEAN SALAD

SERVES: *2* // **PREP:** *15 minutes* // **COOK:** *10 minutes*

This nutrient-dense salad paired with the slight pepperiness of watercress is bat-flipping good. Mung beans are protein- and fiber-filled legumes similar to peas and lentils. Brazil nuts, loaded with the powerful antioxidant glutathione and a favorite of José Bautista's, add a tasty finish.

4 to 5 Brazil nuts

¼ cup cooked green lentils (see page 13)

¼ cup cooked mung beans (see page 13)

½ cup diced bell pepper (red/green/yellow)

2 tablespoons finely diced red onion

2 tablespoons chopped fresh mint

½ teaspoon finely grated peeled ginger root (a Microplane is great for this)

½ teaspoon ground turmeric

½ teaspoon ground coriander

1 tablespoon extra-virgin olive oil

2 tablespoons fresh lime juice

Salt and freshly ground pepper

3 cups watercress or baby arugula

1. Preheat the oven to 375°F.

2. Lay the Brazil nuts on a sheet pan and toast for 8 minutes, until they just begin to brown. Let cool before coarsely chopping. Set aside.

3. In a large bowl, combine the lentils, mung beans, bell pepper, red onion, mint, ginger, turmeric, coriander, olive oil, and lime juice. Season with salt and pepper to taste.

4. Divide the watercress between 2 plates. Divide the lentil-bean mixture over the watercress. Top with the toasted Brazil nuts.

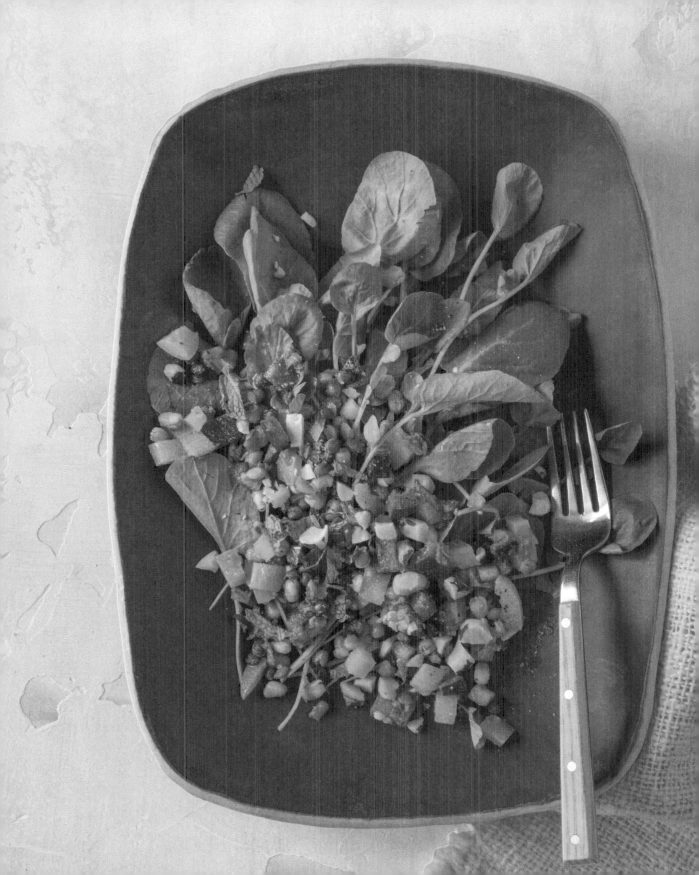

SEARED AVOCADO

SERVES: *2* // **PREP:** *5 minutes* // **COOK:** *10 minutes*

For avocado lovers, this snack is a no-brainer. The punchy flavors of chili powder, cayenne, and cumin are offset by the sweet creaminess of the avocado.

2 tablespoons nuts (e.g., pistachios, almonds, walnuts)

½ teaspoon chili powder

¼ teaspoon ground cumin

¼ teaspoon freshly ground pepper

⅛ teaspoon cayenne

⅛ teaspoon salt

1 avocado, halved and pitted

1½ teaspoons coconut oil

1. Preheat the oven to 375°F.

2. Lay the nuts on sheet pan and toast for 7 to 9 minutes, until they just begin to brown. Let cool, then chop. Set aside.

3. In a small bowl, combine the chili powder, cumin, black pepper, cayenne, and salt. Sprinkle the mixture over the cut sides of the avocado.

4. In an 8-inch nonstick skillet, heat the oil over medium heat. Cook the avocado, flesh-side down, for 2 to 3 minutes, until golden brown.

5. Remove from the heat and let cool slightly. Sprinkle with the nuts. Serve with a spoon for scooping the avocado out of its shell.

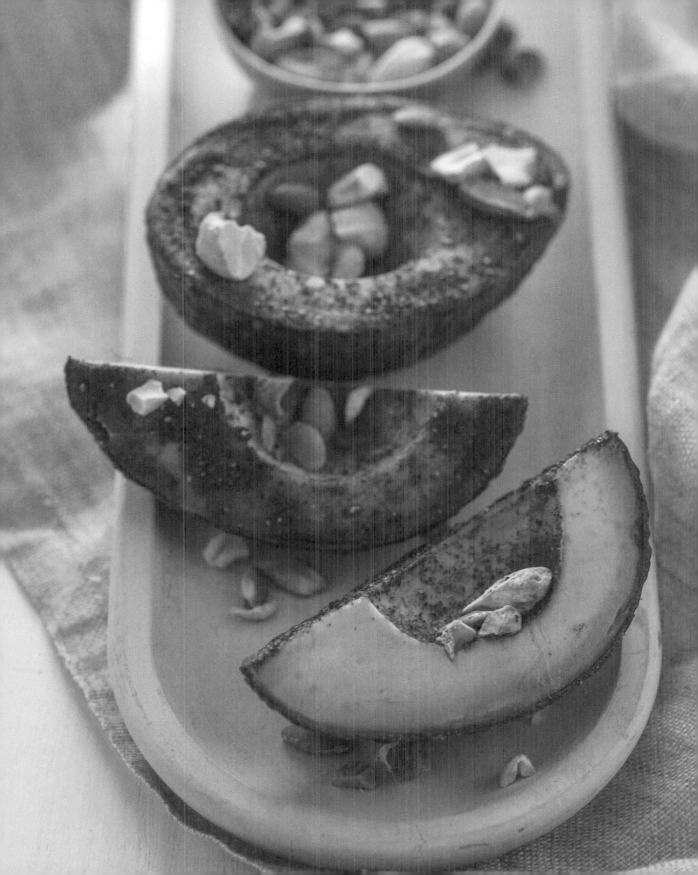

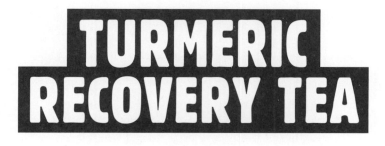

TURMERIC RECOVERY TEA

SERVES: *1* // **PREP:** *10 minutes* // **COOK:** *10 minutes*

Turmeric is the key ingredient that helps reduce inflammation in this soothing tea. Be sure to toss in some black peppercorns to boost its absorption.

3-inch piece of turmeric root, chopped (about ¼ cup)

Peel of lemon (save the fruit for another recipe)

⅛ teaspoon black peppercorns

½ teaspoon raw honey (optional)

In a saucepan over medium heat, bring the turmeric, lemon peel, peppercorns, and 2½ cups water just to a boil and simmer for 7 minutes. Strain and add the honey (if using).

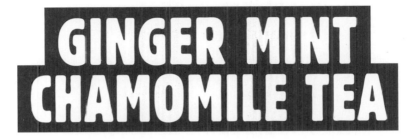

GINGER MINT CHAMOMILE TEA

SERVES: 1 // **PREP:** 5 minutes // **COOK:** 10 minutes

For fans of caffeine-free tea, chamomile combined with mint brings tranquility to your day. The fresh ginger helps boost digestion and your immune system. Sit back and enjoy the healthful benefits of each sip.

2½ cups chamomile tea (see Note)
1½-inch piece of ginger root, chopped
Handful of fresh mint leaves (about ⅓ cup)

In a saucepan over medium heat, bring the tea, ginger, and mint to a low simmer; continue simmering for 8 to 10 minutes. Strain and serve hot.

Note: To make your own chamomile tea, steep 2 tablespoons chamomile tea leaves in 2½ cups boiling water for 5 minutes. Strain out the tea leaves.

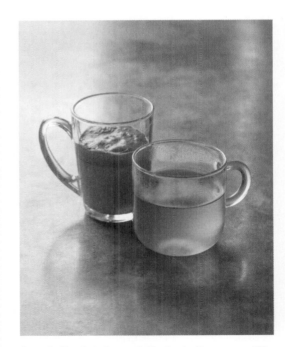

From left: Hot Coconut Mocha Latte, *page 170* (Ian Kinsler); Ginger Mint Chamomile Tea

TROPICAL SMOOTHIE

SERVES: *1* // **PREP:** *15 minutes, plus 2 hours for soaking*

Inspired by José Bautista's Dominican roots, the tropical fruit gives this smoothie great texture and flavor. If you can't find mango or papaya—or if they're out of season—chunks of fruit like grapefruit, orange, or kiwi can easily pinch-hit. Brazil nuts are a great source of selenium, an immune-boosting and stress-fighting mineral.

6 Brazil nuts

1 cup chilled rice milk

¼ cup coarsely chopped mango

¼ cup coarsely chopped papaya

1 banana, broken into pieces

½ passion fruit, flesh scooped out

1. In a small bowl, soak the Brazil nuts in room-temperature water for 2 hours. Strain, rinse, and drain.

2. In a high-powered blender, combine the nuts, milk, mango, papaya, banana, and passion fruit and process until smooth.

▼ TROPICAL
SMOOTHIE

▲ STRAWBERRY KIWI
BANANA SMOOTHIE,

PAGE 87
(CARLOS CORREA)

▲ KITCHEN SINK
SMOOTHIE,

PAGE 141
(ADAM JONES)

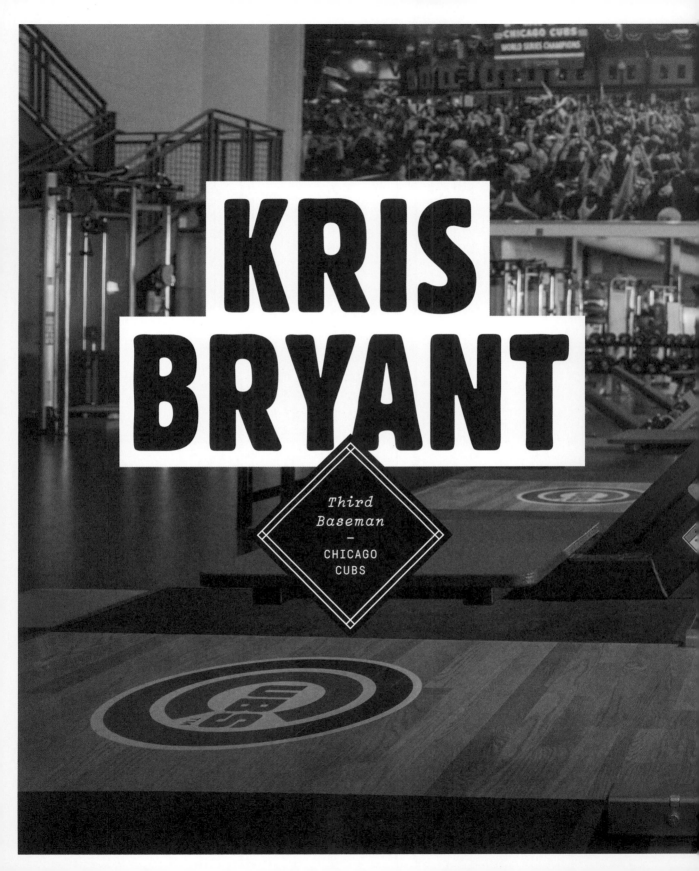

KRIS BRYANT

Third Baseman
—
CHICAGO CUBS

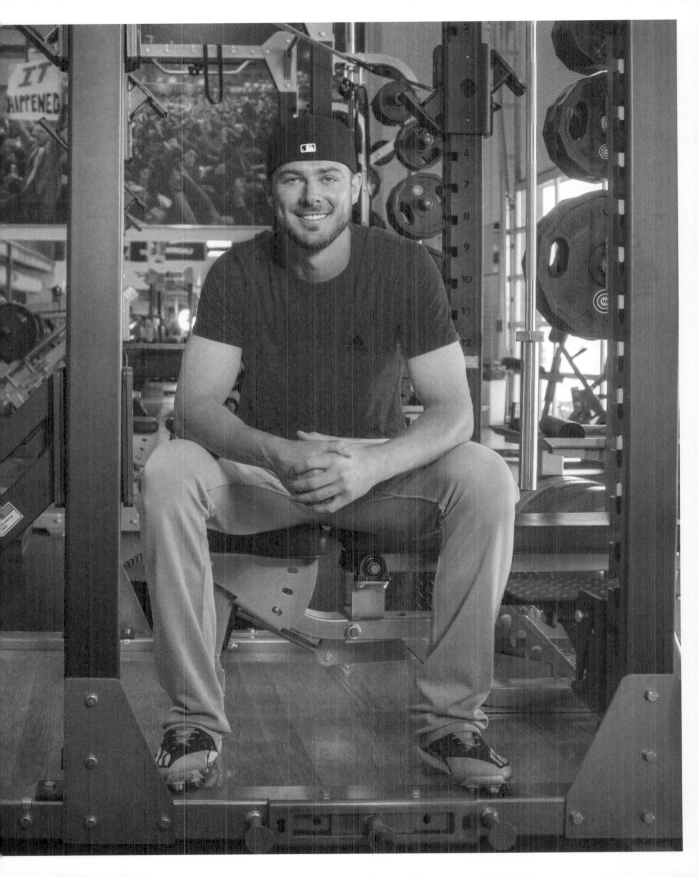

I want to play the game for as long as I can, so if eating right is going to help me do that, I would be a fool not to take advantage. I talk to older guys on the team and hear them say how they wish when they were younger they had all the information we have now about how food helps you perform better. Many of them have said they probably could have played an extra five years if they had changed their diets early on in their careers. And the teams are doing a great job helping us with that too.

Breakfast is the hardest meal for me during the season when we have a night game. Once our game is over, I'll leave the field around 11:30 p.m., get home by midnight, and won't go to sleep for a couple hours; I need to cool down. I watch TV. So I probably sleep until, like, 12:30. For me breakfast sometimes becomes a kind of lunch. In general, breakfast is my favorite meal. I like eggs, breakfast potatoes.

FULL NAME: Kristopher Lee Bryant

HEIGHT/WEIGHT: 6'5", 230 lbs

BORN: January 4, 1992, in Las Vegas, NV

POSITIONS: Third baseman and outfielder

DRAFT: Drafted by the Toronto Blue Jays in the 18th round of the 2010 MLB Draft and the Chicago Cubs in the 1st round (2nd) of the 2013 MLB Draft

HIGH SCHOOL: Bonanza High School (Las Vegas, NV)

COLLEGE: University of San Diego (San Diego, CA)

AWARDS AND RECOGNITION: 2016 World Series Champion; 2x NL All-Star; 2015 NL ROY; 2016 NL MVP; 2016 NL Hank Aaron Award

My ideal lunch is a chicken and rice bowl. Chicken, rice, black beans, avocado, salsa, and no dressing or any of that. Chicken and rice give you plenty of energy. That's my go-to.

My favorite smoothie has strawberry and banana, and then I throw in spinach or kale and make it green. You don't really taste the greens but you know they're good for you. I think the greens open up your blood vessels and get the blood flowing, which is something I never would have known two years ago.

My favorite vegetables are broccoli and zucchini. It's pretty easy to make broccoli taste good—maybe add a little salt to it. And I love spicy seasonings.

During the World Series I ate pretty much the same way I eat during the rest of the year. You never know how you are going to react to a different meal so I keep it fairly consistent. Our team chef does a good job switching things up, but with a similar base—like honey mustard chicken or a Caribbean jerk chicken. It's all organic. We'll occasionally get burgers but all from grass-fed beef.

The biggest difference I have perceived since starting to eat better is how much easier it is to wake up in the morning. Last off-season I would sleep until about 10:30 a.m., and then go work out. This off-season, I only sleep until 8:30 because it's easier to get out of bed.

For me, a healthy snack is a trail mix with things like almonds and peanuts, and maybe I'll throw in a couple of chocolate chips. My other snacks are things like half a wrap or half a salad. I'll have a Philly cheese wrap without the cheese, but with bell pepper and onion. Even in salads, throwing in the peppers makes it a little different, which I love. I never really knew that I liked them. I throw them in anything. And I'm a picky eater.

When I was playing college baseball, we had a team psychologist who taught us visualization as a way to prepare for our games. Everyone was skeptical at first, including me, but seeing the results made it easier to keep doing it. I still use that technique today, as I need it. When you're playing well you don't need it as much because you feel good about yourself. But it's important to do visualization exercises when the slumps come through because

you can close your eyes and go back in time to when you were doing well, to what you were doing and how you felt. It helps you reposition yourself. I take all that into my game preparation. I know it works. Especially in baseball; it's such a tough game. It's built around failures and you need that positive reinforcement to make sure you're mentally prepared, staying healthy, and getting the right amount of sleep. You need to be able to give positive reinforcement to yourself. After a bad game, I find it easier to sleep at night when I can lie down and visualize the next game.

I've learned that you don't have to take the game home with you. Balance is key. Baseball is my job, and I don't want to take my job home. I think you find that peace sitting with friends and family. My wife and I go home and watch TV and try to be normal people in a crazy world. We don't go out or any of that. We think about how lucky we are and are thankful for what we have.

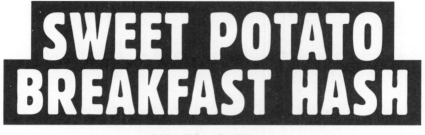

SWEET POTATO BREAKFAST HASH

with Black Beans

SERVES: *2* // **PREP:** *20 minutes* // **COOK:** *15 minutes*

Nutritious sweet potatoes make Kris Bryant's favorite breakfast hash extra tasty. The touch of heat from the habanero will kick-start your day, but be sure to wear gloves when handling it (or use cayenne instead for a milder taste). The maple syrup adds just the right balance of flavor when served at the end over the added earthy black beans.

2 cups diced sweet potato

1 cup diced peeled turnips

2 tablespoons finely diced shallots

1½ teaspoons coconut oil, melted

¼ teaspoon ground cumin

⅛ teaspoon minced seeded habanero pepper or a pinch of cayenne

Salt

1 cup cooked black beans, warm (see page 12)

½ teaspoon pure maple syrup

1 tablespoon chopped scallion greens

2 lime wedges

1. Preheat the oven to 400°F.

2. In a large bowl, toss together the sweet potato, turnips, shallots, oil, cumin, and habanero until well combined. Arrange in a single layer on a baking sheet and bake for about 15 minutes, until the vegetables are golden and tender. Remove from the oven and season with salt to taste.

3. Transfer the hash to 2 bowls. Spoon the black beans in the middle of each bowl and drizzle with maple syrup. Sprinkle scallion greens on top and squeeze a lime wedge over each serving.

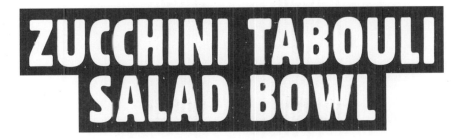

ZUCCHINI TABOULI SALAD BOWL

SERVES: *2* // **PREP:** *25 minutes*

This gluten-free slant on a traditional tabouli is still packed with crunch and loaded with taste. The cannellini beans, an excellent source of protein, make this salad a seriously satiating lunch or dinner.

2 cups diced zucchini

1 cup diced red bell pepper

1 cup chopped fresh flat-leaf parsley

2½ tablespoons fresh lemon juice

2½ tablespoons extra-virgin olive oil

1 cup cooked cannellini beans (see page 12)

Salt and freshly ground pepper

3 cups mixed salad greens

2 tablespoons hemp hearts

¼ teaspoon smoked paprika

1. In a large bowl, combine the zucchini, bell pepper, parsley, lemon juice, and olive oil.

2. Fold in the beans and season with salt and pepper to taste.

3. Divide the mixed greens between 2 salad bowls and add the zucchini tabouli. Top with hemp hearts and a sprinkle of paprika.

CARIBBEAN CHICKEN AND RICE BOWL

SERVES: *2* // **PREP:** *15 minutes, plus marinating time* // **COOK:** *30 minutes*

With just the right balance of heat that is suitable for a wide range of palates, this modern jerk-style chicken is a no-doubter. When handling the habanero, don't forget to wear gloves to protect your skin from the habanero oils.

MARINADE

2 tablespoons chopped onion

2 tablespoons chopped scallion, white and green parts

4 garlic cloves, smashed

1-inch piece of ginger, peeled and chopped (about 2 tablespoons)

2 tablespoons tamari

2 tablespoons ketchup

1 tablespoon fresh thyme leaves

1 tablespoon fresh lime juice

¼ habanero pepper, seeded and coarsely chopped (about 1 teaspoon)

½ teaspoon allspice

1 teaspoon coconut sugar

2 whole bone-in chicken breasts (1 to 1¼ pounds each)

Rice and Vegetables (recipe follows)

1. In a food processor, combine the marinade ingredients and pulse until smooth. Place the chicken breasts in a large baking dish. Coat the chicken with the marinade. Cover with plastic wrap and marinate in the refrigerator for at least 2 hours or up to 24 hours.

2. Preheat the oven to 375°F. Bake the chicken with the marinade until an instant-read thermometer inserted in the thickest part of the meat, not touching the bone, reads 165°F, about 30 minutes. Serve with Rice and Vegetables, spooning any juices from the baking dish over the chicken.

RICE AND VEGETABLES

SERVES: *2* // **PREP:** *20 minutes*

2 cups cooked brown rice (see page 13)

2 cups diced bell peppers

½ cup shredded carrots

¼ cup chopped fresh flat-leaf parsley

1½ tablespoons extra-virgin olive oil

2½ tablespoons fresh lime juice

Salt and freshly ground pepper

In a large bowl, combine the rice, peppers, carrots, parsley, olive oil, and lime juice. Season with salt and pepper to taste and toss well.

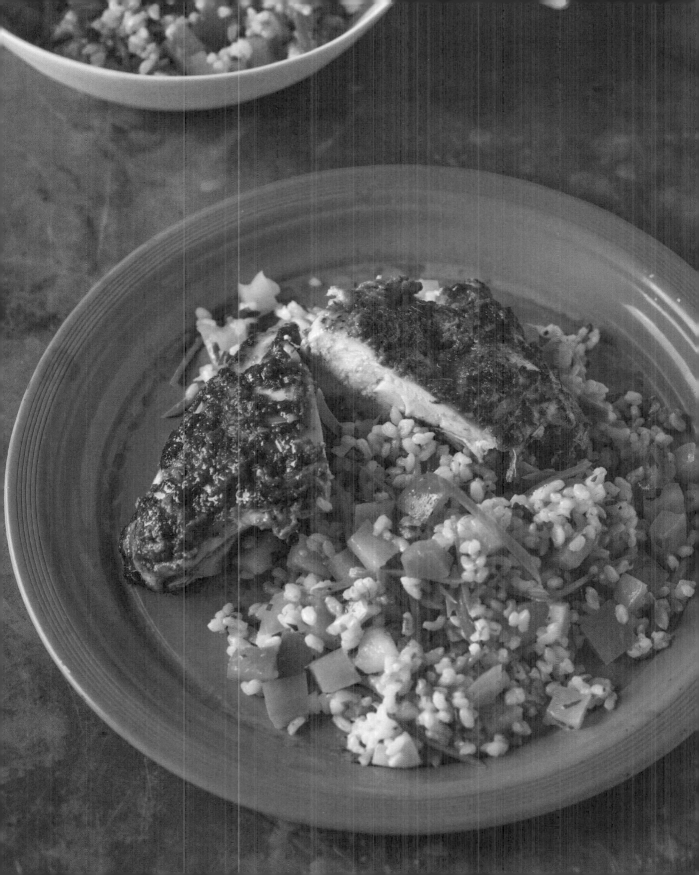

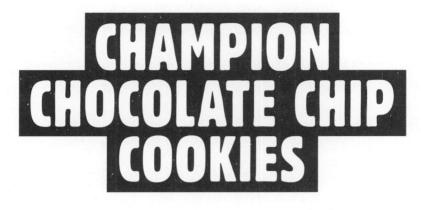

CHAMPION CHOCOLATE CHIP COOKIES

MAKES: *22 cookies* // **PREP:** *5 minutes* // **COOK:** *20 minutes*

The beauty of these gluten-free chocolate chip cookies is that they still have the sweet stuff, only healthier. For a convenient way to always have cookie dough ready to bake, place the raw dough balls side-by-side in an airtight container and keep them in the freezer. When ready to make, simply remove from the freezer, transfer to a baking sheet lined with parchment paper or a silicone mat and bake. Just be sure to add an extra two minutes of baking time for the frozen dough to bake completely.

2 large eggs

¼ cup coconut sugar

2 cups almond flour

2 tablespoons oat flour

**¼ cup mini dark chocolate chips
(sweetened with coconut sugar or stevia)**

¼ teaspoon baking soda

Pinch of salt

2 tablespoons coconut oil, melted

1. Preheat the oven to 375°F. Line 2 baking sheets with parchment paper or a silicone mat.

2. In a large bowl, whisk the eggs and sugar for 2 minutes until pale yellow.

3. In a medium bowl, whisk together the almond flour, oat flour, chocolate chips, baking soda, and salt. Add the dry ingredients to the egg mixture and fold in the melted oil. Mix well, using your hands to evenly incorporate ingredients.

4. Use a #60 scoop or 1-tablespoon measure to portion about 22 cookie dough balls, divided between the prepared baking sheets. Flatten the balls into 1½- to 2-inch rounds by pressing them with the flat bottom of a small glass dipped in water. Bake, alternating the middle rack position halfway through, for about 10 minutes, until the cookies are slightly firm to touch.

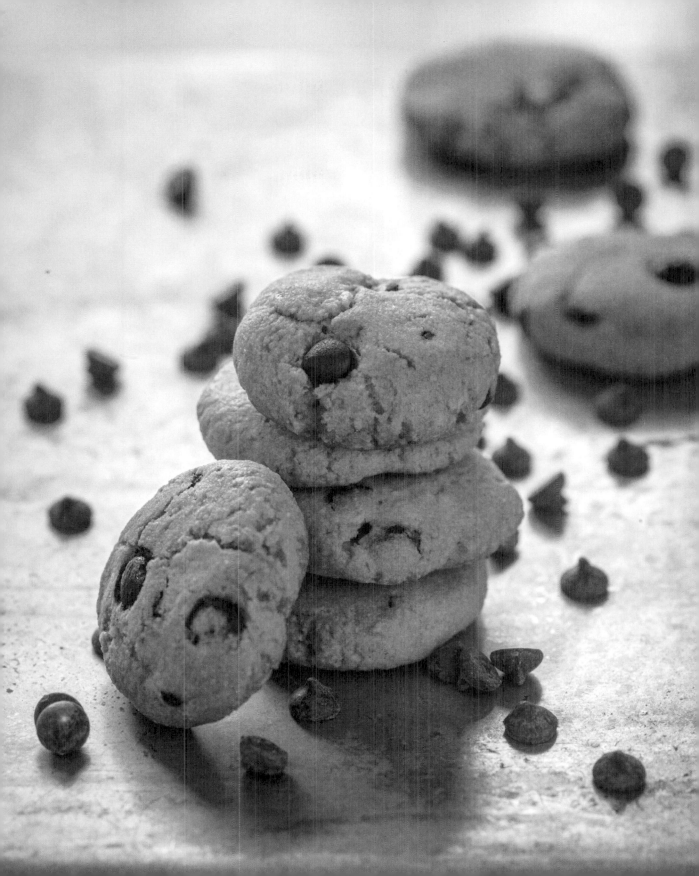

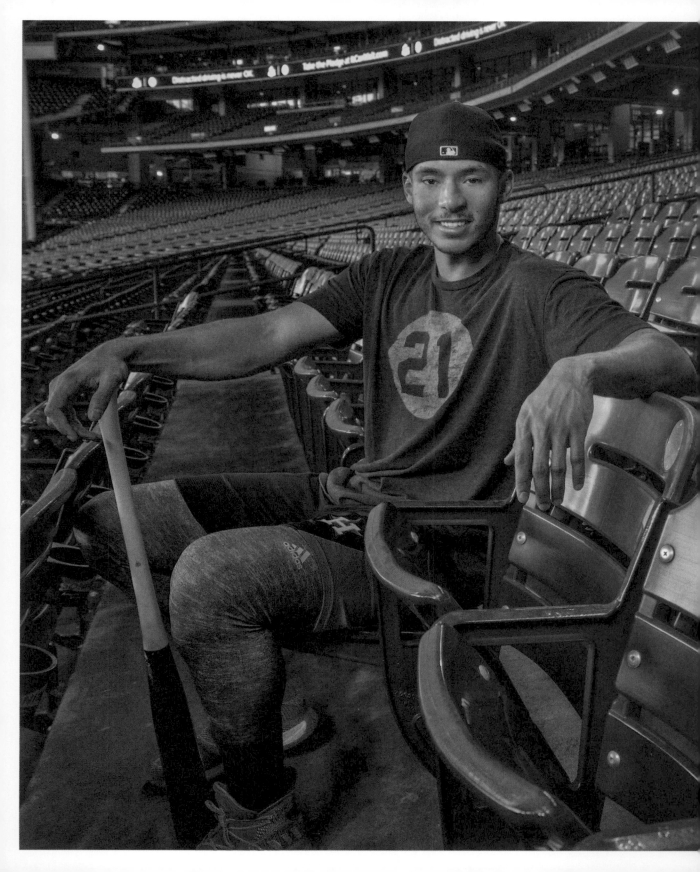

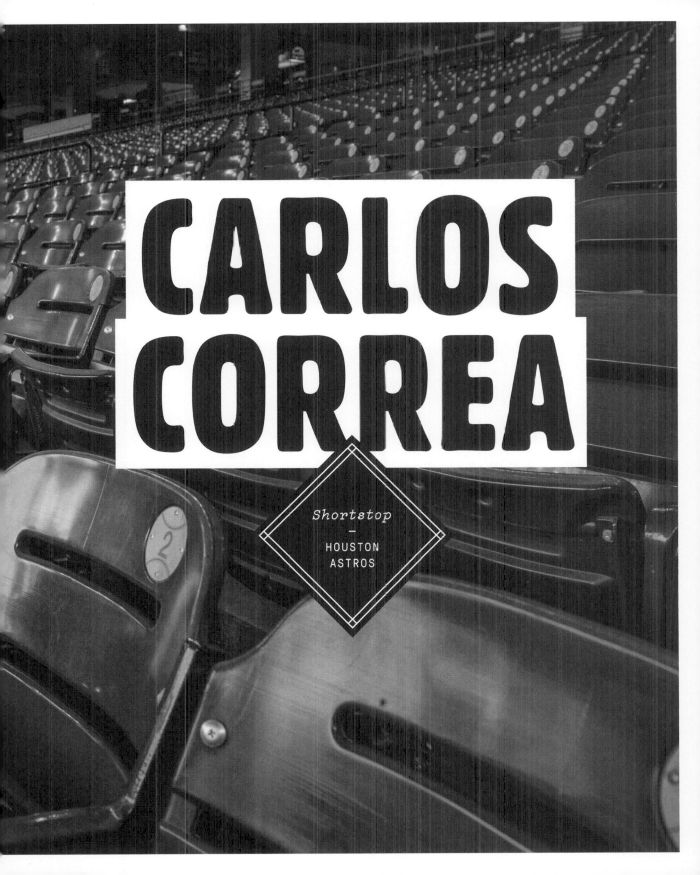

CARLOS CORREA

Shortstop

—

HOUSTON ASTROS

One of the first steps I took to improve my performance was to find a nutritionist during my first year in pro ball. I was seventeen years old. She helped me eat the right way. Being 6 foot 4, I never want to get too heavy. I want to eat well and still be strong and flexible. I want to be able to move around easily. To do that I've got to work hard, I've got to sleep well, and I've got to eat healthy too.

My breakfast routine always includes eggs with ham and a little bit of cheese. I like cheese, but just a little bit. I eat oatmeal and then a Greek yogurt with fruit. And I drink a lot of water. This is my biggest meal of the day.

My favorite fresh juice or smoothie is one that my mom makes for me when I'm home. It has banana, strawberry, mango, and papaya, and she pours in freshly squeezed orange juice and water.

I eat clean snacks like Greek yogurt with granola and fruit, which give me great energy. I avoid fried foods, soda, beer, alcohol, and processed sweets like candy, doughnuts, cookies, and brownies.

Lunch is usually rice and beans with some avocado. Also, I often eat one or two

FULL NAME: Carlos Javier Correa

HEIGHT/WEIGHT: 6'4", 215 lbs

BORN: September 22, 1994, in Ponce, Puerto Rico

POSITION: Shortstop

DRAFT: Drafted by the Houston Astros in the 1st round (1st) of the 2012 MLB Draft

HIGH SCHOOL: Puerto Rico Baseball Academy and High School (Gurabo, PR)

AWARDS AND RECOGNITION: 2017 World Series Champion; 2017 AL All-Star; 2015 AL ROY

pieces of salmon, as I need to eat a lot to stay energized throughout the day. Then for dinner I'll have chicken and red-skinned potatoes with broccoli on the side. I love eating rice. I could eat rice with every meal, and red beans.

I started eating healthier for my career because I wanted to get better on the field, and in order to do that I had to sacrifice some of the foods I like. Now I eat a lot of fresh vegetables, including broccoli and carrots, which I never used to like. I also wasn't big into fish at first, but now I eat salmon and mahi-mahi all the time.

I am careful not to eat a lot of carbohydrates before I go to bed. I eat more protein instead. I notice I have much more energy when I wake up.

I want to play shortstop until I'm forty! I started eating well at a young age—hopefully I can keep doing it, since eating well prevents injuries.

Baseball is what drives me, but I also kayak a lot and I swim. I like going to the ocean—I'm from Puerto Rico so the ocean is in my backyard. I just like being active.

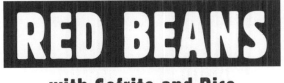

RED BEANS

with Sofrito and Rice

SERVES: *2* // **PREP:** *15 minutes* // **COOK:** *5 minutes*

The peppers give this dish a lot of pop, but the avocado and broccoli cool down the heat while adding to the hearty flavors. If you're pepper-shy you can switch them out for a milder bell pepper instead.

1 tablespoon coconut oil

½ cup minced mixed peppers (such as ½ medium seeded poblano, ½ small seeded serrano, 1 small seeded red fresno)

3 tablespoons minced yellow onion

2 teaspoons minced garlic

2 cups cooked red kidney beans (see page 12)

2 tablespoons chopped fresh cilantro

Salt and freshly ground pepper

2 cups cooked short-grain brown rice, warm (see page 13)

Avocado and Broccoli (recipe follows)

1. In a medium saucepan, melt the coconut oil over medium heat. Add the peppers, onion, and garlic and cook, stirring, for 3 to 4 minutes, until soft. Toss in the kidney beans and cook until heated through, stirring constantly.

2. Remove from the heat and fold in the cilantro. Season with salt and pepper to taste. Divide the bean mixture and rice between 2 bowls and top with avocado and broccoli.

AVOCADO AND BROCCOLI

SERVES: *2* // **PREP:** *10 minutes* // **COOK:** *5 minutes*

2 cups broccoli florets

1 avocado, cut into chunks

1 tablespoon sliced scallion, white and green parts

2 tablespoons fresh lime juice

Salt and freshly ground pepper

1. In a saucepan fitted with a steamer basket, bring 1 inch of water to a boil. Put the broccoli in the basket, cover, and steam for 1½ minutes.

2. In a medium bowl, combine the broccoli, avocado, scallion, and lime juice. Season with salt and pepper to taste.

GRILLED MAHI-MAHI

with Carrot-Ginger Rice

SERVES: *2* // **PREP:** *20 minutes* // **COOK:** *10 minutes*

Ginger and turmeric help transform a simple dish into the ultimate palate-pleaser. For a quick and easy way to get finely grated carrots, just use the small tear-shaped holes on a box grater to get the most finely grated carrots.

1½ teaspoons coconut oil

2 skinless mahi-mahi fillets (4 ounces each)

3 cups chopped bok choy

¾ cup finely grated carrot

2 tablespoons thinly sliced scallions, white and green parts

1½ tablespoons fresh lemon juice

1 tablespoon extra-virgin olive oil

1 teaspoon finely grated peeled ginger root

⅛ teaspoon ground turmeric

2 cups cooked brown rice, warm (see page 13)

Salt and freshly ground pepper

1. In a nonstick skillet, heat the coconut oil over medium-high heat. Sear the fish on one side until golden brown, about 3 minutes. Lower the heat to medium. Turn the fish and cook until opaque and cooked through, 2 to 4 minutes, depending on thickness. Transfer to a plate and cover to keep warm.

2. Add the bok choy and a couple drops of water to the skillet and cook, stirring, until just wilted, about 12 seconds.

3. In a large bowl, combine the carrot, scallions, lemon juice, olive oil, ginger, and turmeric.

4. Add the rice and bok choy to the bowl and toss until well combined. Season with salt and pepper to taste. Divide between 2 plates and place the fish on top.

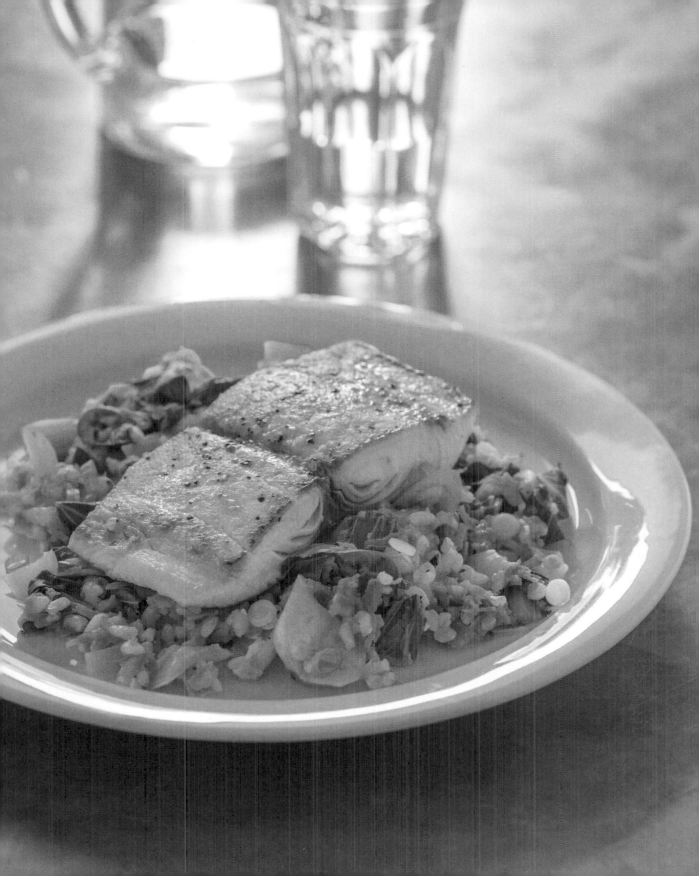

ADOBO RICE CAKES

SERVES: *2* // **PREP:** *15 minutes* // **COOK:** *10 minutes*

Inspired by Carlos Correa's Caribbean roots, these rice cakes couldn't be easier to make as a quick snack. They are infused with wonderful adobo flavors such as onions, garlic, oregano, and citrus.

1 cup cooked short-grain brown rice (see page 13)

1 cup cooked millet (see page 13)

2 tablespoons minced shallot

2 teaspoons minced garlic

1 teaspoon grated orange zest

½ teaspoon dried oregano

¾ teaspoon ground cumin

1 tablespoon chopped fresh cilantro

1 tablespoon thinly sliced scallion

½ teaspoon salt

¼ teaspoon freshly ground pepper

1 tablespoon coconut oil

1. In a food processor, blend the rice, millet, shallot, garlic, zest, oregano, and cumin until it begins to form a dough, 1 to 2 minutes. Transfer to a mixing bowl and stir in the cilantro, scallion, salt, and pepper. Shape into 6 cakes (about ¼ cup each).

2. Heat the oil in a nonstick skillet over medium heat. Cook the cakes until golden brown on each side, 7 to 9 minutes total.

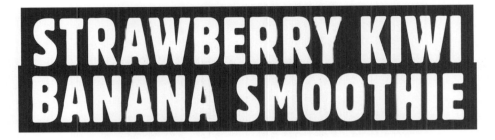

STRAWBERRY KIWI BANANA SMOOTHIE

SERVES: 1 // **PREP:** *15 minutes*

Coconut water is a great electrolyte replacement, especially after a tough workout. The super freshness of kiwi in this smoothie (pictured on page 69) is what knocks it out of the park.

1 cup quartered hulled strawberries
½ cup chopped peeled kiwi
1 banana, broken into chunks
½ cup chilled raw coconut water

In a high-powered blender, combine the strawberries, kiwi, banana, and coconut water and process until smooth.

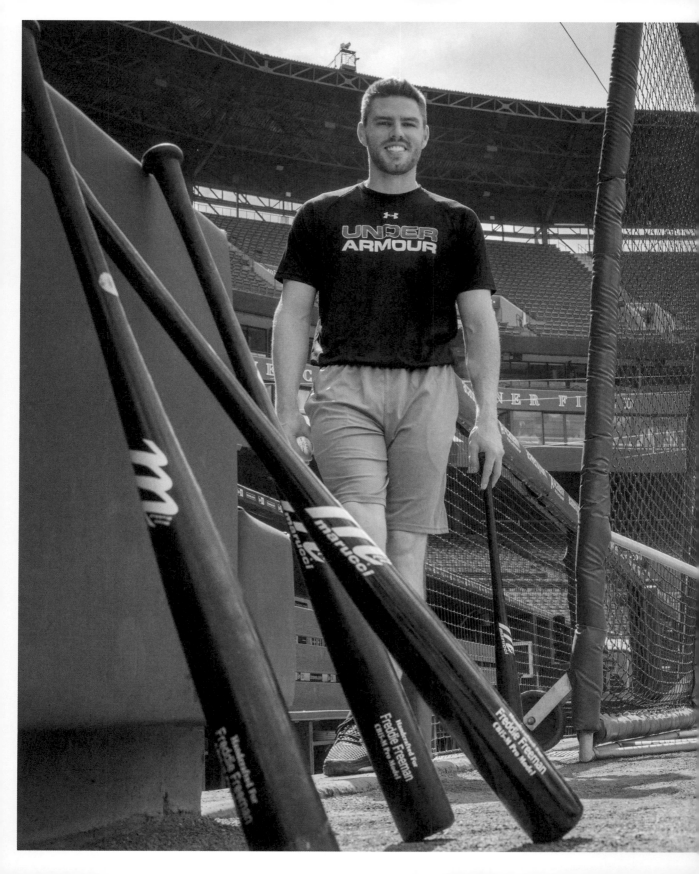

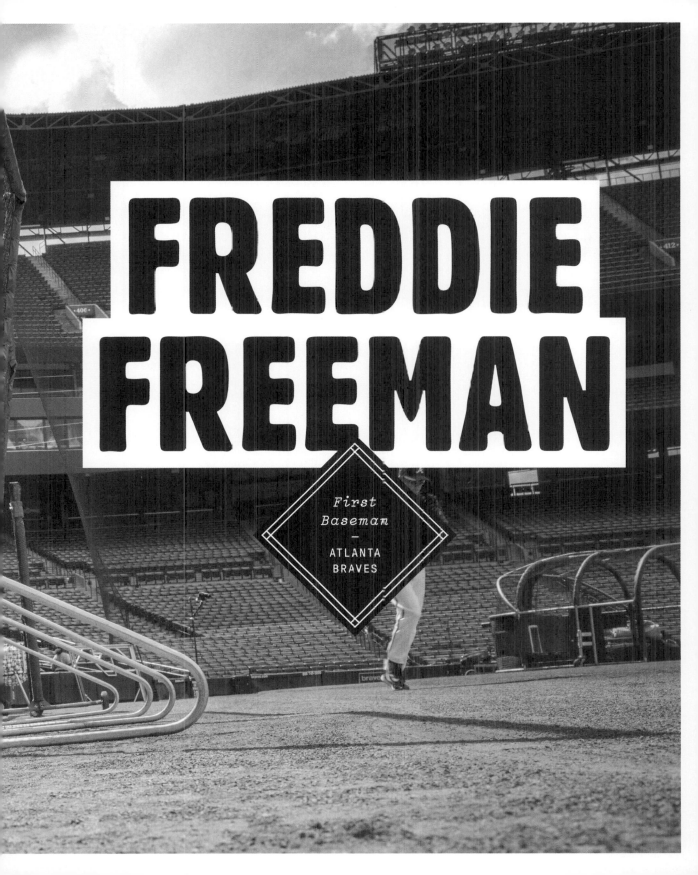

FREDDIE FREEMAN

First Baseman
—
ATLANTA BRAVES

My former teammate Dan Uggla motivated me to start eating well. When Dan was in his early thirties, he started eating better and went gluten-free. I watched what he ate, I watched how he worked out, and it just rubbed off on me. My dad also motivated me. He was diagnosed with heart disease. At one point he weighed more than three hundred pounds and has since lost a hundred pounds.

One of the biggest changes I made in my diet was to cut back on sugar. I ate a lot of sugary cereal when I was growing up. I stopped that. I eat a lot of fruits now instead, especially berries. I started to see everybody around me eating healthy food and I saw how their bodies changed. I wanted to change mine too. I also cut back on salt and gluten.

I noticed a connection between food and performance when I first got into the big leagues at the age of twenty. I was a very soft 245 pounds. I came to camp overweight and was overweight for probably the first two years of my professional career. I was a lot bigger than I am now and I didn't feel well. My right knee started to hurt, things started to feel like they would break down from playing 162 games with all that weight.

FULL NAME: Frederick Charles Freeman

HEIGHT/WEIGHT: 6'5", 220 lbs

BORN: September 12, 1989, in Fountain Valley, CA

POSITION: First baseman

DRAFT: Drafted by the Atlanta Braves in the 2nd round of the 2007 MLB Draft

HIGH SCHOOL: El Modena High School (Orange, CA)

AWARDS AND RECOGNITION: 3x NL All-Star; 2018 NL Gold Glove Award; hit for the cycle on June 15, 2016

I wasn't where I needed to be in my career or with my body. It took me a while to make food changes. It's been a five-year process, but I'm almost where I want to be.

Eggs give me energy to work out in the morning. After my workout, I usually make a protein shake with raw whole-grain oats, bananas, peanut butter, organic milk, and ice. I blend it up and it tastes amazing! For breakfast I eat something with eggs, like quiche or an omelet.

I used to drink a lot of milk and soda. I also ate a lot of sugary cereals. Now, I always drink water and I just started trying fresh cold-pressed juices. I also drink a lot of tea, like English breakfast tea in the morning or a jasmine tea with honey in it. My wife's family is from England, so I got into tea.

One of the biggest changes I've made to my diet is to eat more home-cooked meals. My mother passed away when I was ten years old, and my dad didn't really know what to do about food. We had a couple of home-cooked meals here and there but mostly it was fast food. I didn't have that upbringing of eating well, and it took me a long time to figure it out. I still don't know it all, but I am doing a lot better than I have in the past.

"*After my workout, I usually make a protein shake with raw whole-grain oats, bananas, peanut butter, organic milk, and ice. I blend it up and it tastes amazing!*"

My biggest meal of the day is lunch—something like a high-protein organic enchilada. I eat a lot of grilled chicken. Lemon-grilled chicken breasts are my favorite with a lot of carrots, broccoli, and other vegetables. For dinner I usually have chicken or maybe a piece of grilled salmon with miso on it. I also recently discovered that I really like quinoa.

The biggest improvement I've experienced from changing my diet is increased energy throughout the day. I don't feel as blah when I get up in the morning. In the past, when I had a big meal at night, I would feel lethargic when I woke up, and sleep in until nine or ten in the morning. I took that as a sign that my body wasn't in the best shape. You get used to eating healthy, and if you don't, your body reacts. So it's been an interesting change for me, but a wonderful one that I needed in my life.

The best wellness advice I've received is to stick to your plan and don't veer from it. Now I go to the grocery store and see all the desserts and they look so good, but I just keep walking. I can have dessert once in a while, but the days of having it all the time are over. I know I'll be better off later on in life. I'd like to see my grandkids grow up.

Besides eating smart, my support for living smart comes from family. I got married in 2014, and my wife has made a big impact on me. She met me when I was at 245 pounds and loved me. She helped me. We now have a son, and I'd like to be able to live long enough to help him and play with him through all the years like my dad was able to do with me.

"CHEESY" SPINACH AND BROCCOLI FRITTATA

SERVES: *4* // **PREP:** *15 minutes* // **COOK:** *20 minutes*

Freddie Freeman likes to start his day with eggs, but this breakfast dish is so versatile, you could also pair it with a salad for lunch or dinner. The key to making the perfect frittata is a seasoned cast-iron skillet.

2 cups chopped broccoli florets

8 large eggs

3 tablespoons nutritional yeast

Pinch of crushed red pepper flakes (optional)

Salt and freshly ground pepper

1½ teaspoons coconut oil, melted

½ cup diced onion

2 cups chopped baby spinach

Handful of basil, torn

1. In a saucepan fitted with a steamer basket, bring 1 inch of water to a boil. Put the broccoli in the basket, cover, and steam for 1½ minutes. Remove from the basket and allow to cool.

2. Preheat the oven to 400°F.

3. In a medium bowl, whisk the eggs with the nutritional yeast, red pepper flakes (if using), and salt and pepper to taste. In a 9-inch ovenproof nonstick skillet or seasoned cast-iron skillet, heat the oil over medium heat. Add the onion and cook, stirring occasionally, for about 4 minutes, until golden brown.

4. Add the broccoli and egg mixture to the skillet and stir with a rubber spatula for 1 to 2 minutes until the eggs begin to set. Remove from the heat. Fold in the spinach and basil and use the spatula to smooth the surface. Bake for 12 to 14 minutes, until the eggs are set. Let the frittata cool for a few minutes before cutting into 4 wedges.

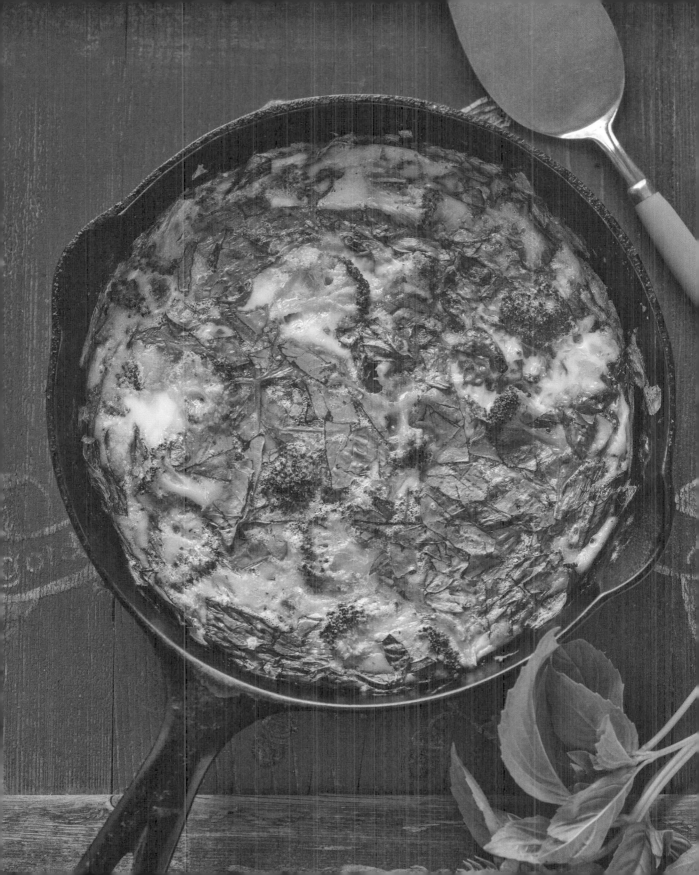

TURKEY AND ZUCCHINI ENCHILADAS

SERVES: *2* // **PREP:** *25 minutes* // **COOK:** *30 minutes*

Zucchini provides a different take on traditional corn enchiladas. This vegetable version is so delicious even Freddie Freeman would agree. If pressed for time, you can make the sauces ahead, refrigerate, and assemble the ingredients the next day. Any extra cheese sauce also goes nicely with the Quinoa Burger Stack on page 52.

1½ teaspoons coconut oil, plus more for the dish

12 large (7½ x 2 inches) zucchini sheets (from 1 large zucchini), shaved thin lengthwise on a mandoline

¼ cup finely chopped yellow onion

8 ounces ground turkey (dark and white meat)

6 pitted kalamata olives, thinly sliced

½ teaspoon dried oregano

½ teaspoon ground cumin

¼ teaspoon chili powder

Salt

3 cups baby spinach

Tomato Sauce (recipe follows on page 96)

"Cheese" Sauce (recipe follows on page 96)

1. Preheat the oven to 375°F.

2. Grease a shallow casserole dish (about 10 x 8 x 1 inch) with a dab of oil. Arrange 6 zucchini slices so that the ends start in the middle of the dish horizontally and overhang one long edge of the dish (overlapping them slightly; see photo, opposite). Repeat with the remaining 6 slices on the opposite side of dish, with the ends meeting in the middle. This will allow you to wrap the overhanging slices around the filling.

3. In a large skillet, heat 1½ teaspoons oil over medium heat. Add the onion and cook, stirring, until golden brown, 3 to 4 minutes. Add the turkey and cook, breaking it up with a wooden spoon, until cooked through, about 5 minutes. Stir in the olives, oregano, cumin, chili powder, and salt to taste. Layer the spinach on top, cover, and cook until just wilted, about 2 minutes. Toss the ingredients to combine.

4. Spoon the filling across the middle of the layered zucchini. Fold over the zucchini ends, first on one side and then the other, tucking them up and over the filling to enclose it. Ladle tomato sauce around the enchiladas and bake for 15 minutes. Drizzle with ¼ cup of the "cheese" sauce and bake for another 5 minutes.

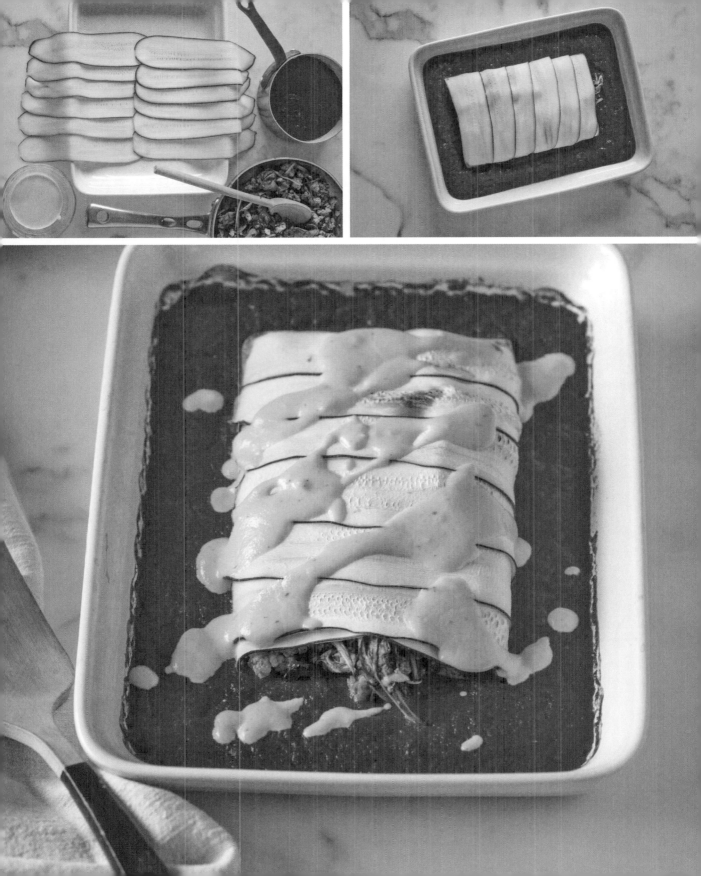

TOMATO SAUCE

MAKES: *1 cup* // **PREP:** *10 minutes* //
COOK: *35 minutes*

1 red bell pepper

Coconut oil

1 cup drained canned plum tomatoes, ½ cup
    tomato juice reserved

Pinch of coconut sugar

Salt and freshly ground pepper

1. Rub the pepper with just a dab of oil and
roast over an open flame (or in the oven; see
Note), turning every so often, until the entire
surface is blackened. Place in a bowl and cover
to allow the pepper to steam and soften for
about 15 minutes. Peel the pepper but leave a
few specks of burnt skin for flavor. Discard the
seeds but do not run under water. Chop.

Note: If you can't cook over an open flame,
preheat the oven to 450°F. On the top
rack close to the heat source but without
touching, roast the oiled pepper for 10 to
15 minutes, turning every 5 minutes, until
the skin begins to blister and blacken.
Prepare the pepper as in step 1.

2. In a small saucepan over medium-low
heat, combine the roasted pepper, tomatoes,
reserved tomato juice, and sugar. Simmer,
stirring and breaking up the tomatoes, for
about 20 minutes, until most of the liquid has
evaporated.

3. Transfer the sauce to a high-powered
blender and process, scraping down the sides
occasionally, until very smooth. Season with
salt and pepper to taste.

"CHEESE" SAUCE

SERVES: *4* // **PREP:** *5 minutes* //
COOK: *2 minutes*

½ teaspoon coconut oil

1 teaspoon minced garlic

½ cup raw cashews

1½ teaspoons fresh lemon juice

2 teaspoons nutritional yeast

⅛ teaspoon ground cumin

Pinch of crushed red pepper flakes
    (optional)

1. In a small skillet, heat the oil over medium
heat. Add the garlic and cook, stirring
constantly, until golden, about 1 minute.

2. Transfer the garlic to a high-powered
blender along with the cashews, ⅓ cup water,
lemon juice, nutritional yeast, cumin, and
pepper flakes, if using. Blend until smooth.
Store any extra sauce in the refrigerator in an
airtight container for up to 3 days.

STRAWBERRY LEMON QUINOA LOAF

SERVES: *6–8* // **PREP:** *10 minutes* // **COOK:** *30 minutes*

With a hint of sweetness and a satisfying texture, this delightful loaf is a huge hit for good reason. Enjoy a slice or two as a snack or breakfast treat with tea. The quinoa and flaxseed are both great sources of fiber.

2 tablespoons plus 2 teaspoons coconut oil, melted, plus more for the pan

2 cups cooked white quinoa (see page 13)

1½ cups chopped hulled strawberries, plus more for garnish

2 large eggs, lightly beaten

1 cup oat flour

3 tablespoons ground flaxseeds

2 tablespoons coconut sugar

½ cup fresh lemon juice

½ teaspoon salt

1. Preheat the oven to 375°F.

2. Use a dab of oil to grease a 1½-quart glass loaf pan.

3. In a food processor, blend the quinoa with the 1½ cups strawberries for 20 seconds. Transfer to a large bowl and stir in the eggs, flour, flaxseeds, sugar, 2 tablespoons of the oil, lemon juice, and salt until well combined.

4. Scrape the batter into the loaf pan and bake for 30 to 35 minutes, until firm and cooked through. Cool before cutting into 6 to 8 slices. Heat the remaining 2 teaspoons oil in a large skillet and toast the slices until golden brown, about 2 minutes per side. Top with additional strawberries.

MISO LEMON SHRIMP

with Kale Slaw

SERVES: *2* // **PREP:** *20 minutes* // **COOK:** *5 minutes*

Miso brings a wonderful sweet and salty flavor combo to grilled shrimp. Another key to this beautiful and tasty dish is letting the kale slaw stand for ten minutes before serving. This allows the flavors to combine and transforms the slaw into a sweeter mixture, which adds another delectable dimension to the grilled shrimp.

8 ounces (10 to 15) medium shrimp, shell on, deveined

2 teaspoons coconut oil

1 teaspoon white miso

1 tablespoon fresh lemon juice

½ teaspoon grated shallot

Salt

Kale Slaw (recipe follows)

1. Using a sharp paring knife, cut along the backside of each shrimp shell. Remove the vein that runs along the back of the shrimp, preferably without rinsing. Dry the shrimp well with paper towels.

2. In a medium skillet, heat the oil over medium heat. Add the shrimp, and cook, turning halfway through, until just opaque, about 4 minutes total. Transfer to a plate. When cool enough to handle, remove the shells.

3. In a medium bowl, combine the miso, lemon juice, and shallot and season with salt to taste. Add the shrimp and toss to coat. Place the shrimp on top of the slaw and drizzle the remaining sauce over top.

KALE SLAW

SERVES: *2* // **PREP:** *20 minutes*

1 cup thinly sliced, curly kale, tough ribs removed

1 cup shaved Savoy cabbage

3 tablespoons thinly sliced radishes

2 tablespoons thinly sliced scallions, white and green parts

1 tablespoon fresh lemon juice

1½ teaspoons unseasoned rice wine vinegar

1½ teaspoons extra-virgin olive oil

Salt and freshly ground pepper

In a large bowl, combine all the ingredients. Season with salt and pepper to taste. Let stand for 10 minutes before serving.

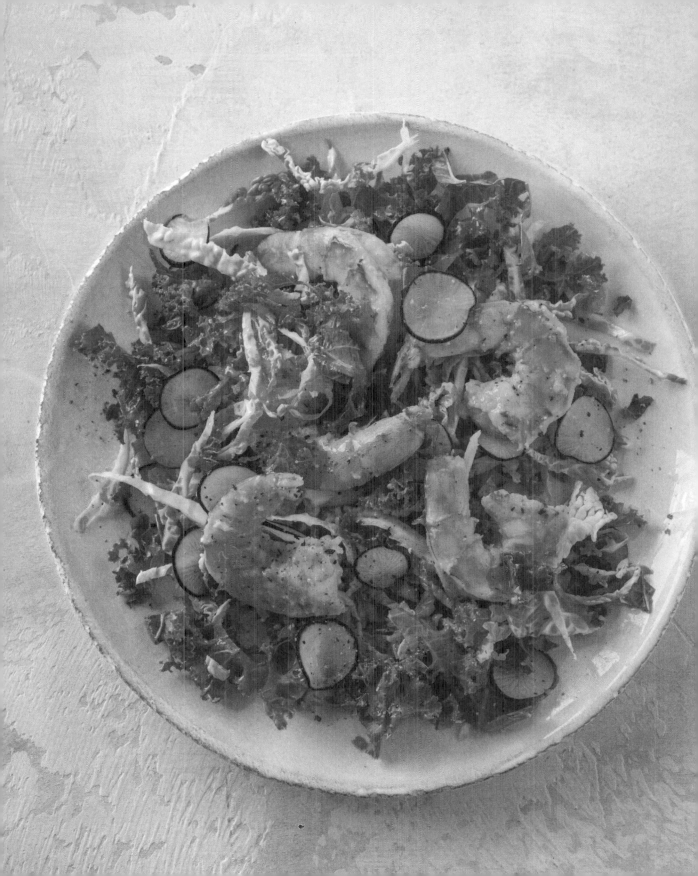

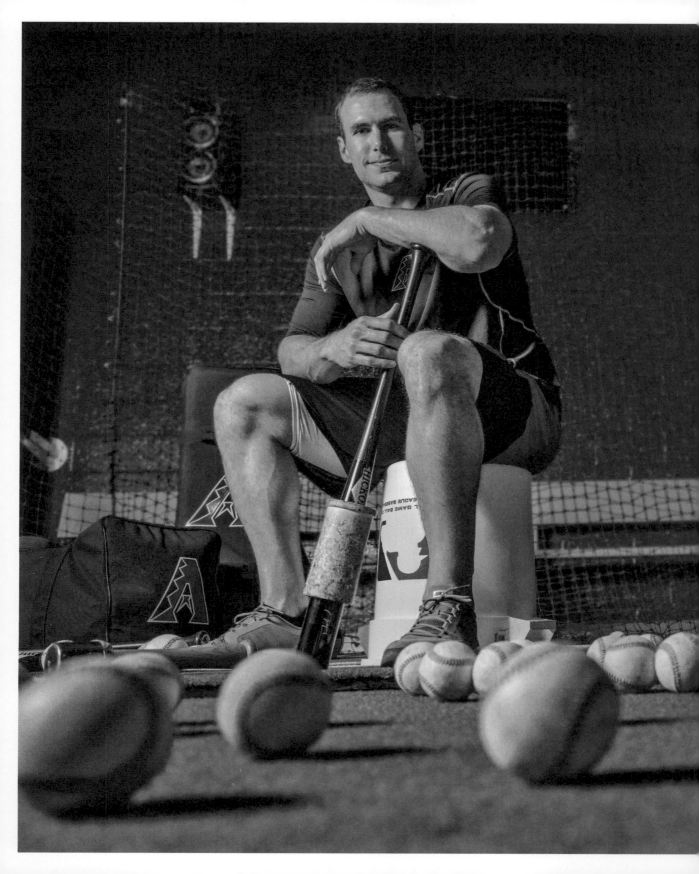

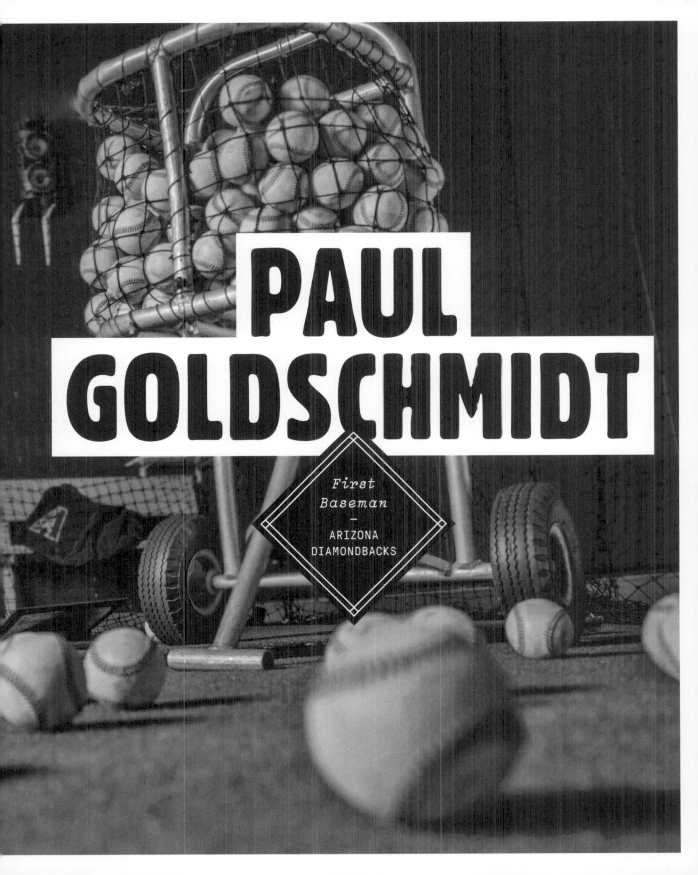

PAUL GOLDSCHMIDT

First Baseman
—
ARIZONA
DIAMONDBACKS

My motivation for eating well started after I was drafted. I went to rookie ball and started playing seven days a week compared to the four I had been playing in college. I had a good year, but my body went through a big adjustment once I started playing daily. I was tiring easily and knew I needed to build up my endurance. During the off-season I decided to lose weight. I was drafted at 245 pounds and lost twenty pounds. I started to feel a lot better. Once I got to the big leagues, the training staff promoted the benefits of healthy eating. I felt the difference and performed better on the field. Eating better helped prepare me for the long season and prevent injury.

My eating philosophy is simple: Eat well. I'm not perfect about it, but that's part of the plan. If I'm too strict with myself, there'll come a time when I get a huge craving for something that's not healthy and I'll cave. It's good if I crave something and then eat it in a small portion. That helps stop the craving from escalating into a much bigger slip-up.

If I'm going to eat sugar, I prefer that it come from fruit, and I try to eat fruit in the morning along with a couple of eggs. I also try to throw something green in there. Spinach is the easiest thing to add to meals.

FULL NAME: Paul Edward Goldschmidt

HEIGHT/WEIGHT: 6'3", 225 lbs

BORN: September 10, 1987, in Wilmington, DE

POSITION: First baseman

DRAFT: Drafted by the Los Angeles Dodgers in the 49th round of the 2006 MLB Draft and the Arizona Diamondbacks in the 8th round of the 2009 MLB Draft

HIGH SCHOOL: The Woodlands High School (The Woodlands, TX)

COLLEGE: Texas State University (San Marcos, TX)

AWARDS AND RECOGNITION: 6x NL All-Star; 3x Gold Glove Award; 4x NL Silver Slugger Award; 2013 NL Hank Aaron Award; 2013 NL home run leader; 2013 NL RBI leader

Some of my favorite vegetables are broccoli, green beans, butternut squash, and Brussels sprouts. For a snack I often have bell peppers or celery with hummus, instead of chips and salsa. I also like avocados and avocado toast for snacks.

In the off-season we make a lot of juices at home. My favorite fresh juice is made with spinach and kale, ice, and some berries. I make a big container of it.

I try to listen to what my body needs after a game or workout. So in the off-season my biggest meal of the day is lunch, since I work out in the morning. During the season it's probably either breakfast or a meal after the game, depending on when the game ends.

Dinner during the season includes protein—that's after a game to replenish energy. If it's a really long and strenuous game, I'll include carbs like potatoes or rice, but if it's a shorter game I stay away from them and eat more green vegetables. During the off-season I love to

> *"The best way to get started when you want to eat well is to just keep it simple. Eat more vegetables and less bad stuff. Understand what you put in your body, what you drink and eat, how you breathe, the way you sleep."*

cook—I have a bunch of cookbooks I follow for recipes. My wife and I are fortunate to be able to buy grass-fed beef. We buy a portion of a cow, and the fish we eat is wild-caught. And I buy organic chicken.

When it comes to food shopping, I read the ingredients list on everything I buy. Grocery stores are awesome now with organic food offerings. If you're comparing two products at the grocery store and one has twelve ingredients and the other two, the one with two ingredients is going to be better for you. I try to stay away from ingredients with weird names. It's a very simple approach but it's an easy way to see which product is better for you.

The best way to get started when you want to eat well is to just keep it simple. Eat more vegetables and less bad stuff. Understand what you put in your body, what you drink and eat, how you breathe, the way you sleep. If you spend more time and even money on the food you eat, you'll spend less time being sick and at the doctor's office. But you have to put in the work.

AVOCADO TOAST
with Spinach Pesto

SERVES: *1* // **PREP:** *10 minutes* // **COOK:** *5 minutes*

Avocado toast is still a fan favorite. As Paul Goldschmidt's go-to snack, it is even better with a layer of tasty spinach pesto and a sprinkling of pumpkin seeds and hemp hearts. Hemp hearts, or shelled hemp seeds, are a quick and effortless protein source.

2 (½-inch-thick) slices of Big League Bread (page 34)

2 tablespoons Spinach Pesto (recipe follows)

1 ripe avocado, cut into chunks

2 lemon wedges

Salt and freshly ground pepper

1 tablespoon pumpkin seeds

1 tablespoon hemp hearts

1. Toast the bread. Spread 1 tablespoon Spinach Pesto on each slice. Divide the avocado chunks between the toast slices.

2. Squeeze a lemon wedge over each slice, season with salt and pepper to taste, and top with the pumpkin and hemp hearts.

SPINACH PESTO

SERVES: *6* // **PREP:** *5 minutes*

4 ounces baby spinach

3 tablespoons extra-virgin olive oil

1 tablespoon nutritional yeast

2 teaspoons fresh lemon juice

½ teaspoon minced garlic

Pinch of crushed red pepper flakes

Salt and freshly ground pepper

In a food processor, combine all the ingredients except the salt and pepper and pulse until smooth. Season with salt and pepper to taste.

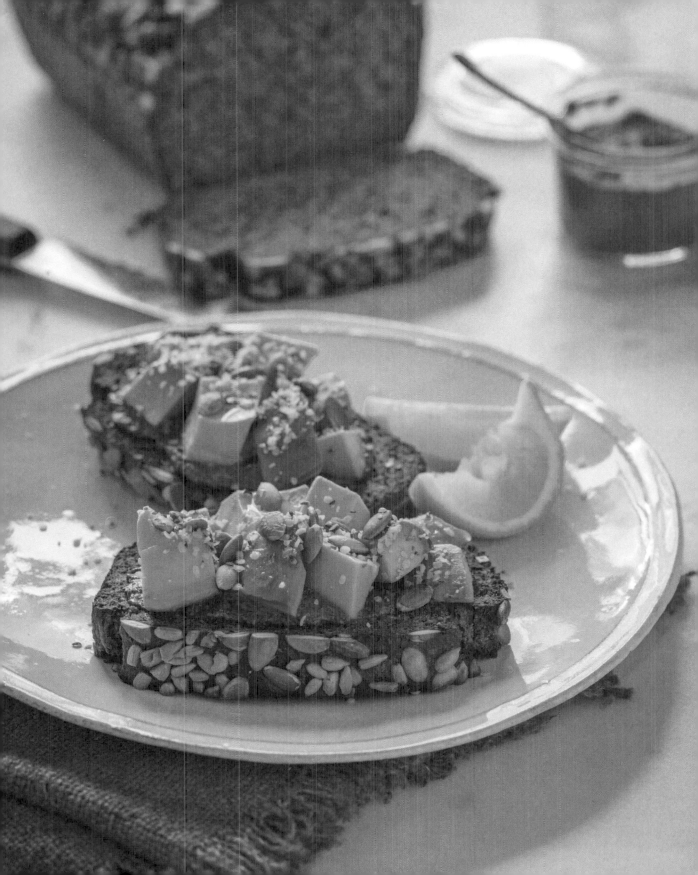

LEMON BUTTERNUT "RISOTTO"

SERVES: *2* // PREP: *20 minutes* // COOK: *20 minutes*

This fresh take on traditional risotto is much easier to whip up. The blended butternut squash creates a creamy texture, and using precooked rice means less time in the kitchen and more time to watch the game.

3 cups peeled, seeded, and diced butternut squash

2½ teaspoons coconut oil, melted

¼ cup chopped yellow onion

1 tablespoon chopped garlic

2 cups cooked short-grain brown rice (see page 13)

1 tablespoon fresh lemon juice

1 teaspoon finely chopped fresh rosemary

Salt and freshly ground pepper

Roasted Asparagus (recipe follows)

1. Preheat the oven to 400°F. Toss 1 cup of the squash with 1 teaspoon of the oil and spread on a sheet pan in a single layer. Roast, stirring once, for about 15 minutes, until golden brown and tender.

2. Meanwhile, in a medium saucepan, heat the remaining 1½ teaspoons oil over medium-high heat. Add the onion and garlic and cook, stirring, until golden brown, about 2 minutes. Add the remaining 2 cups butternut squash and 1½ cups water. Bring to a boil. Cover and simmer until the squash is very tender, about 12 minutes. Remove from the heat and allow to cool for 5 minutes.

3. Puree the squash mixture in a blender. Scoop the puree back into the saucepan. Fold in the rice, lemon juice, rosemary, and reserved roasted squash and season with salt and pepper to taste. Simmer, stirring, for 3 minutes. Divide between 2 bowls and top with the asparagus.

ROASTED ASPARAGUS

SERVES: *2* // PREP: *5 minutes* // COOK: *10 minutes*

½ pound asparagus, trimmed

1 teaspoon coconut oil, melted

Salt and freshly ground pepper

1 teaspoon fresh lemon juice

¼ teaspoon grated lemon zest

1. Preheat the oven to 400°F.

2. Toss the asparagus with the oil and season with salt and pepper to taste. Spread in a single layer on a sheet pan and roast until tender, about 10 minutes, depending on thickness. Sprinkle with the lemon juice and zest.

SPICY CREOLE HUMMUS

SERVES: *4* // **PREP:** *5 minutes*

Adding Creole seasonings to chickpea hummus gives it a burst of zesty flavor. This is the ideal snack to accompany your favorite raw veggies.

1½ cups cooked chickpeas (see page 12)

3 tablespoons extra-virgin olive oil

3 tablespoons fresh lemon juice

1 tablespoon tahini

1 small garlic clove

⅛ teaspoon cayenne

¼ teaspoon dried oregano

¼ teaspoon Old Bay seasoning

¼ teaspoon salt

In a high-powered blender, combine the chickpeas, oil, lemon juice, tahini, garlic, cayenne, oregano, Old Bay, and salt with ⅓ cup water and process until smooth, 1 to 2 minutes. Serve with raw veggies, such as carrots, cucumber, celery, and radishes, for dipping.

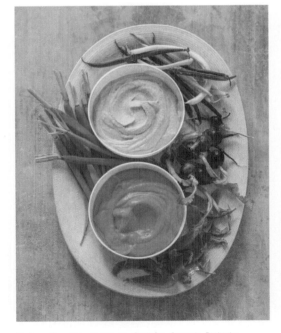

Spicy Creole Hummus (top); Sweet Potato Hummus, page 219 *(Noah Syndergaard)*

FLAT-IRON STEAK

with Bitter Greens and Brussels Sprouts

SERVES: 2 // **PREP:** 30 minutes // **COOK:** 15 minutes

For steak lovers, this full-flavored meal is insanely delicious. The meat is best cooked medium rare to medium to bring out the deep, rich taste and texture. The lemon and olive oil are more readily absorbed when tossed with the hot vegetables, creating the perfect harmony of flavors. Any remaining juices from the meat can be drizzled over the salad as a warm dressing.

½ teaspoon smoked salt

¼ teaspoon Old Bay seasoning

¼ teaspoon freshly ground pepper

8 ounces grass-fed flat-iron steak (½ to ¾ inch thick)

1½ teaspoons coconut oil

2 cups halved Brussels sprouts

2 cups chopped trimmed dandelion greens

1 cup diced bell pepper

½ teaspoon grated garlic

2 tablespoons fresh lemon juice

1 tablespoon extra-virgin olive oil

Pinch of crushed red pepper flakes

Salt

1. In a small bowl, combine the smoked salt, Old Bay, and pepper. Rub the mixture over both sides of the steak and let rest at room temperature for 10 to 20 minutes.

2. In a medium cast-iron skillet, heat the coconut oil over medium-high heat and begin to sear the steak. Once the meat begins to brown, reduce the heat to medium and continue to sear on both sides until the steak reaches the desired doneness (about 8 minutes total for medium). Let the steak rest for 5 minutes before slicing into two portions.

3. In a large saucepan over medium heat, bring ¾ cup water to a boil. Add the Brussels sprouts, cover, and cook until tender, 3 to 4 minutes. Remove from the heat and place the dandelion greens on top of the sprouts. Cover and allow the steam to wilt the greens for 30 seconds to 1 minute.

4. Drain the Brussels sprouts and greens and immediately place in a large bowl. Add the bell pepper, garlic, lemon juice, olive oil, and red pepper flakes. Season with salt to taste. Divide the vegetables between 2 plates and serve with the steak over top.

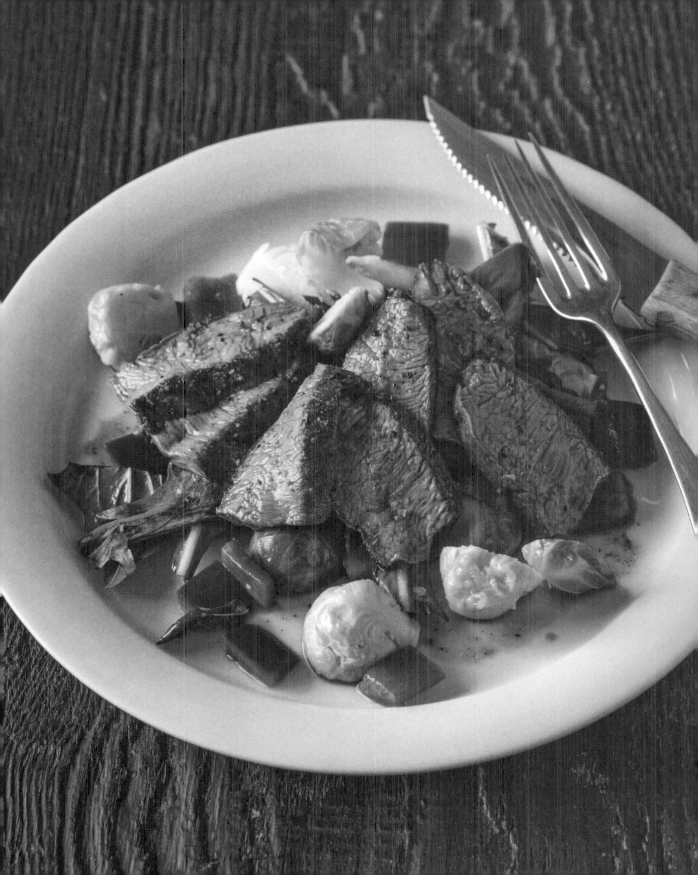

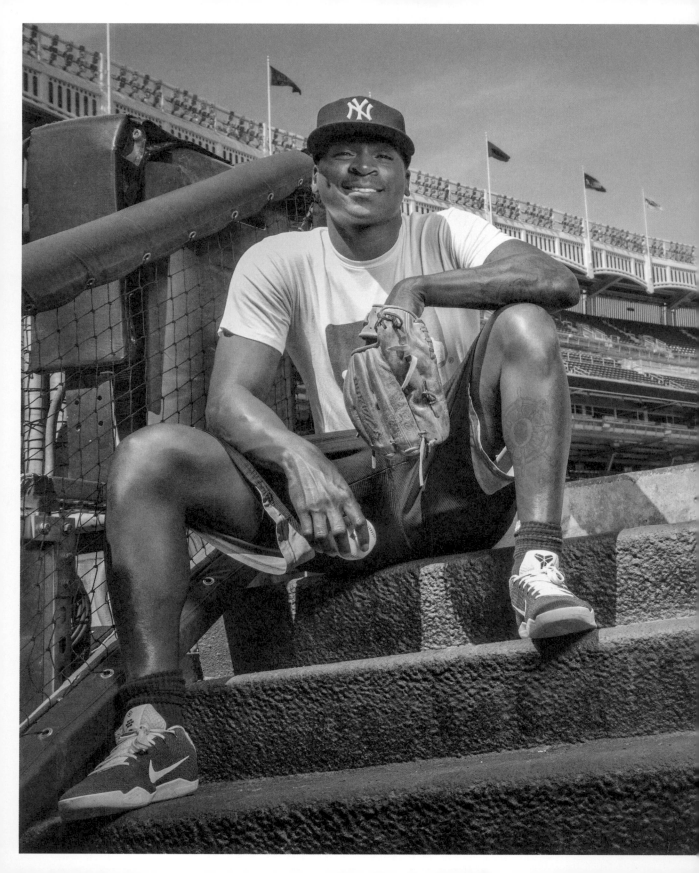

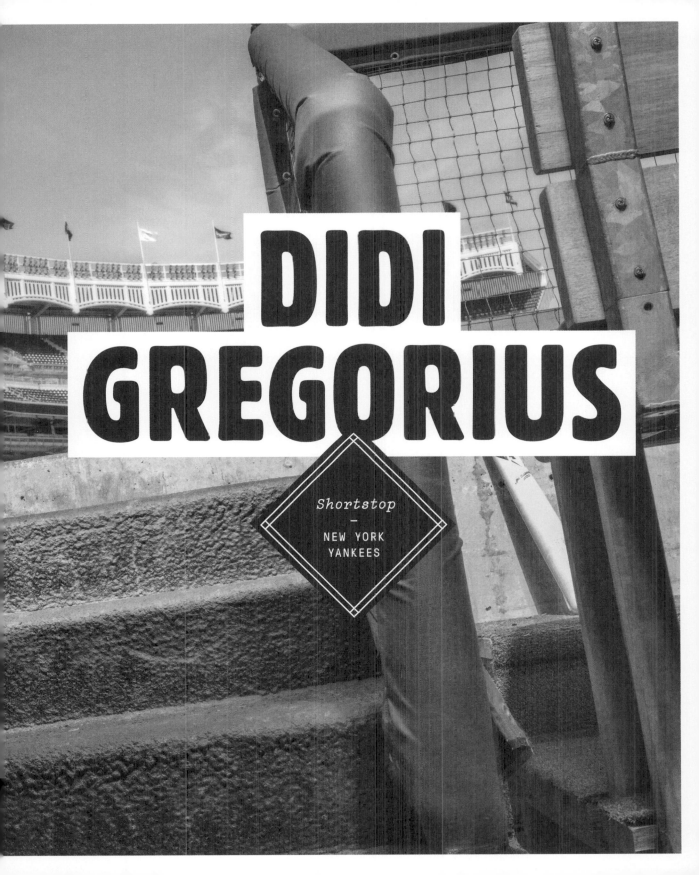

DIDI GREGORIUS

Shortstop
—
NEW YORK
YANKEES

Back in Spring Training in 2010 I was feeling really tired, and I knew something was off. Your body lets you know when something isn't right. Every time I ate red meat, it never felt good in my stomach. Sometimes I would even get sick. I had some tests done. To eliminate the problem, I had to cut out red meat. I don't eat red meat at all anymore. For at least a month I was a vegetarian to get everything under control. Now, I've been eating mostly fish and chicken, which is what I love. I am from Curaçao, and that's what I eat most of the time anyway.

My typical breakfast is egg whites and potatoes. Once in a while I'll have a yogurt.

My favorite fruit is strawberries, but they have to be all-natural, fresh, and organic from a farm stand. And melon too. My favorite green vegetables are asparagus, green beans, and broccoli, and I recently discovered that I also like spinach. I prefer eating my greens instead of juicing them.

My biggest meal of the day is my pregame meal, which is steamed rice with either salmon or chicken. Almost every day I also do a fresh fruit smoothie before the game. Sometimes I blend pineapple, strawberry, and kiwi, or kiwi, banana, and mango, or just mango

FULL NAME: Mariekson Julius Gregorius

HEIGHT/WEIGHT: 6'3", 205 lbs

BORN: February 18, 1990, in Amsterdam, Netherlands

POSITION: Shortstop

SIGNED: As an undrafted free agent in 2007

AWARDS AND RECOGNITION: Won the 2011 IBAF Baseball World Cup and was knighted, along with his teammates, in Curaçao

or strawberry. I mix the fruit with almond milk and a little bit of ice.

For energy on the field, I drink a lot of water to stay hydrated because without a lot of water, my body isn't going to function right. Once in a while before a game, I'll have dark chocolate, almonds, or pistachios. They help give me energy throughout the game.

Back home I grill fish for dinner all the time. For example, when I cook salmon, I put honey and lemon on top, and then grill it. Or I cook chicken. Some guys ask why I only eat chicken and fish, and I explain that this is all my body can take. But I prepare the chicken and fish in a variety of ways. My favorite fish is the one I get back home. I don't know what it would be called here, but back home it's red fish, or as we call it, *pisca cora*.

I like photography and drawing because they keep me calm and let my mind get creative. I like going to beaches when I'm home, and swimming. It helps with muscle recovery and works the tiny muscles. And I relax with my family most of the time. I always try to be myself, be humble, and do things the right way.

The Game of Eating Smart

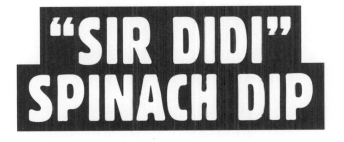

"SIR DIDI" SPINACH DIP

SERVES: *2* // **PREP:** *10 minutes* // **COOK:** *5 minutes*

Impress your guests with this delish dairy-free spinach dip. Nutritional yeast is the star ingredient; it gives the dip a subtle nutty, cheesy flavor.

1 teaspoon coconut oil

1 tablespoon chopped shallots

1 garlic clove, smashed

½ cup cooked cannellini beans (see page 12)

1 tablespoon fresh lemon juice

1 tablespoon extra-virgin olive oil

1½ teaspoons nutritional yeast

Pinch of crushed red pepper flakes

1½ cups packed chopped baby spinach

Salt and freshly ground pepper

1. In a small skillet, heat the coconut oil over medium heat. Add the shallots and garlic and cook, stirring, until golden brown, 3 to 4 minutes.

2. Transfer to a food processor along with the beans, lemon juice, olive oil, nutritional yeast, and red pepper flakes and pulse until smooth, scraping down the sides with a spatula as needed. Add the spinach and pulse until evenly incorporated, 20 seconds. Season with salt and pepper to taste and pulse again.

3. Serve with raw vegetables, such as carrots, cucumbers, celery, and radishes.

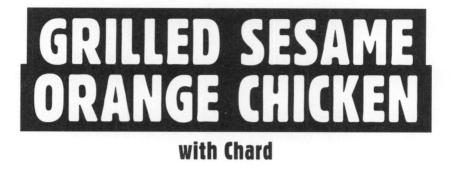

GRILLED SESAME ORANGE CHICKEN

with Chard

SERVES: *2* // **PREP:** *15 minutes, plus marinating time* // **COOK:** *20 minutes*

This chicken dish requires little prep, and marinating the chicken the night before is a huge time saver. The steamed chard is a flavorful contrast, but kale, collards, or escarole work well too.

Peel from 1 orange, coarsely chopped (reserve the fruit for another use)

4 garlic cloves, smashed

2 tablespoons toasted sesame oil

½ teaspoon salt, plus more to taste

¼ teaspoon freshly ground pepper, plus more to taste

2 whole bone-in chicken breasts (about 1 to 1¼ pounds)

1½ teaspoons coconut oil, melted

2 tablespoons toasted sesame seeds

1½ tablespoons fresh lemon juice

2 teaspoons raw honey

3 cups chopped Swiss chard (any color), tough stems removed first

1. In a heavy-duty resealable plastic bag, combine the orange peel, garlic, 1 tablespoon of the sesame oil, ½ teaspoon salt, and ¼ teaspoon pepper. Add the chicken and massage the mixture onto the chicken breasts. Refrigerate for at least 1 hour or up to 24 hours.

2. In a small bowl, stir together the sesame seeds, lemon juice, remaining 1 tablespoon sesame oil, honey, and additional salt and pepper to taste. Set aside.

3. Preheat a grill to medium-high heat and brush the grates with the coconut oil. Remove the chicken from the bag, discarding the garlic and orange peel if desired. Lay the chicken, skin-side down, on the hot grill and cover. Sear the chicken on one side for 7 to 9 minutes, until golden brown and crispy. Flip the chicken and cook for 10 to 12 minutes more, until the internal temperature reaches 165°F at the thickest end of the breast, avoiding the bone. Remove from heat and let rest for 5 minutes.

4. In a saucepan fitted with a steamer basket, bring 1 inch of water to a boil. Put the chard in the basket, cover, and steam until just wilted, 15 to 20 seconds. Remove from heat and season to taste with salt.

5. Remove the chicken from the bone and cut crosswise into ¼-inch-thick slices. Divide the chard between 2 plates, top with chicken, and drizzle the reserved lemon sesame sauce over top.

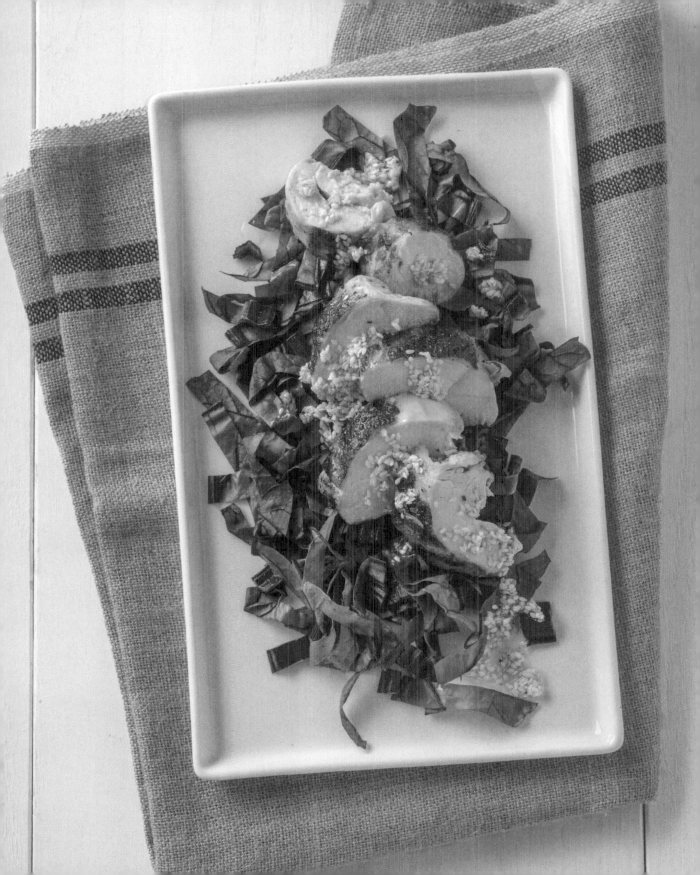

SUPERFOOD TRUFFLES

MAKES: *10 truffles* // **PREP:** *10 minutes*

Get all your essential nutrients plus mega deliciousness in just one bite. These highly addictive truffles incorporate two powerful ingredients: detoxifying chlorella and anti-aging, anti-inflammatory royal jelly.

¼ cup almond butter

2 tablespoons unsweetened cacao powder

2 tablespoons raw honey

1 teaspoon chlorella powder

1 teaspoon chia seeds

½ teaspoon royal jelly

1 tablespoon plus 1 teaspoon hemp hearts, for coating

1. In a medium bowl, combine all of the ingredients except the hemp hearts. Use the back of a spoon to drag the ingredients across the bottom of the bowl to mix well.

2. Once the ingredients are fully incorporated, use a #100 scoop (slightly under 1 tablespoon) or your hands to portion the mixture into ten 1-inch balls.

3. Roll the balls in the hemp hearts. The truffles will keep in the refrigerator for up to 3 months wrapped in wax paper and stored in an airtight container. If refrigerated, remove and serve at room temperature.

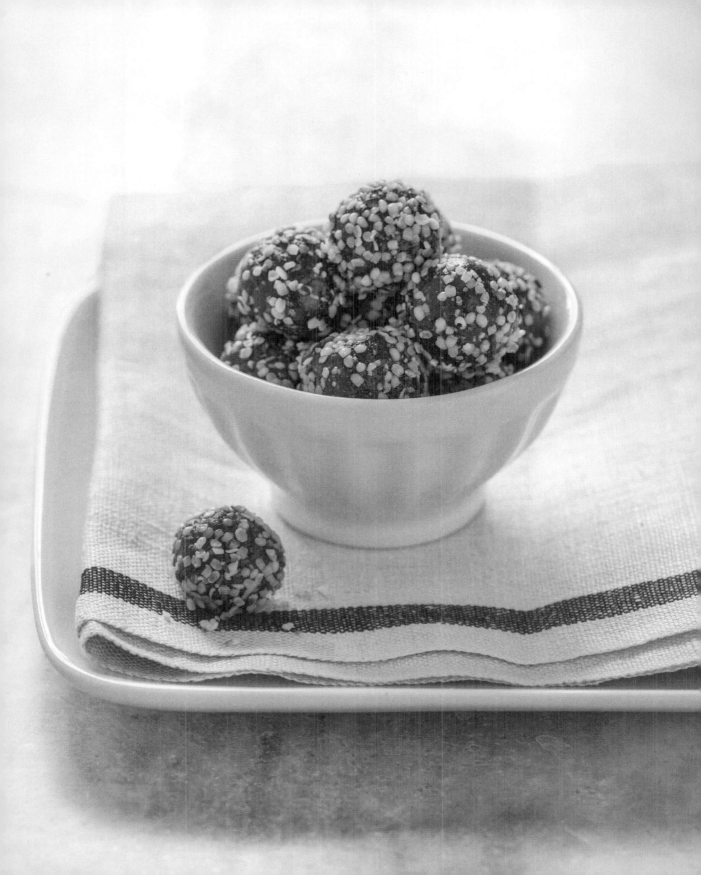

COCONUT YOGURT

with Pistachio Granola

SERVES: *2* // **PREP:** *5 minutes*

Young Thai coconut meat is the key ingredient in this creamy yogurt. Older coconuts have a hairy protective husk on the outside and the meat is more solid and firm. Whole young Thai coconuts are always wrapped in plastic and located in the refrigerator section of most supermarkets. They can be cut open to scoop out the soft, fleshy meat. And some specialty grocers stock prepackaged coconut meat in the frozen food section; simply let it thaw in the refrigerator overnight.

2 cups young Thai coconut meat, thawed if frozen

¼ cup fresh lemon juice

Probiotic powder from 4 probiotic capsules

⅔ cup Pistachio Granola (recipe follows)

In a high-powered blender, blend the coconut meat, lemon juice, probiotic powder, and 3 tablespoons water until smooth. Divide the coconut yogurt between 2 bowls and top each with about ⅓ cup of the granola. The yogurt will keep for up to 4 days in an airtight container in the refrigerator.

PISTACHIO GRANOLA

SERVES: *4* // **PREP:** *5 minutes* // **COOK:** *15 minutes*

1 tablespoon honey

1 tablespoon coconut oil

1 cup coarsely chopped pistachios

¼ cup chopped dried papaya or dried pineapple

¼ cup dried blueberries

1. Preheat the oven to 325°F. Line a baking sheet with a nonstick silicone mat.

2. In a small saucepan over low heat, warm the honey and oil until they blend when you swirl the pot. Remove from the heat and mix in the nuts. Using a flexible spatula, scrape the mixture onto the silicone mat and spread evenly.

3. Bake until the nuts are browned and crisp, stirring occasionally, about 15 minutes. Remove from the oven and immediately mix in the dried fruit.

4. Let the granola cool to room temperature on the baking sheet. Crumble into the desired size pieces and use for topping yogurt or oatmeal. Store any extra granola in the refrigerator in an airtight container for up to 6 weeks.

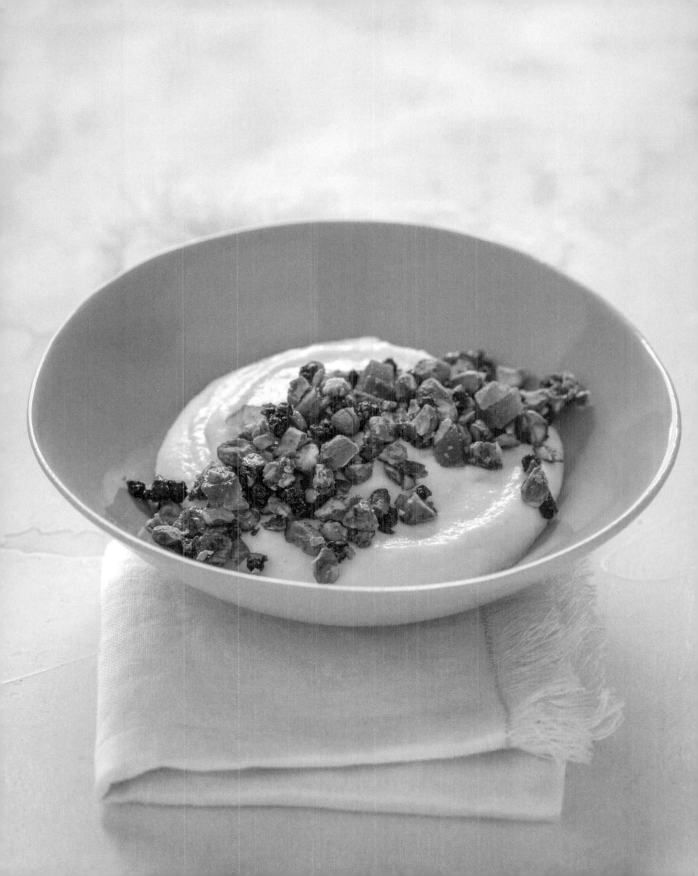

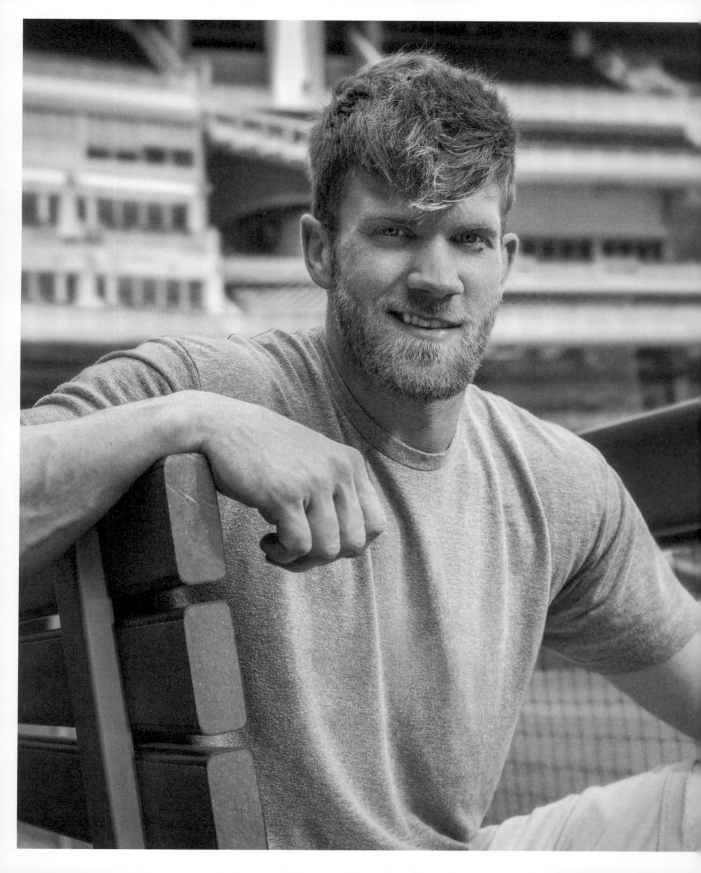

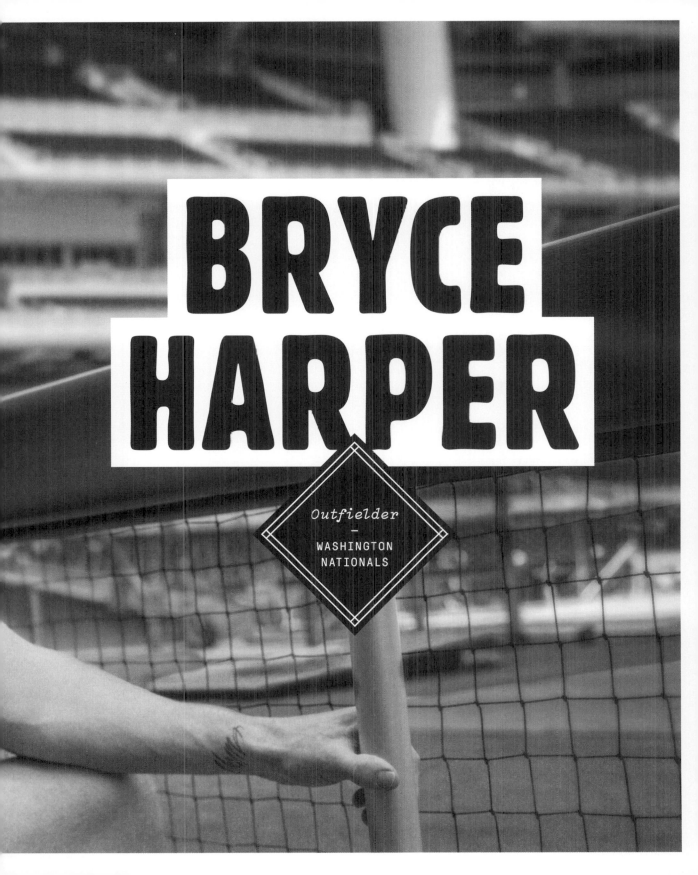

BRYCE HARPER

Outfielder
—
WASHINGTON
NATIONALS

When I was growing up my mom had a home-cooked meal for us every single night. She was my earliest motivation for eating smart—I was blessed to have her cook for me.

I went gluten-free because it just made me feel better and healthier. I was cautious about it when I started, but the longer I went without gluten, the better I felt. The biggest difference is my energy level, which is through the roof. I feel great every day.

My biggest meal is breakfast—I crush it. My go-to breakfast is scrambled eggs with chicken and avocado.

When I'm on the road for away games, I look for restaurants that are farm-to-table or vegan. Even though I'm not a vegan, there are a lot of good vegan places with great food. I'll have a steak or chicken later, so I still get that protein. I enjoy trying new and different things.

Dehydration gets into every single nerve, deep into your system, so you have to keep replenishing. I drink a gallon of water a day—half of it in the morning and the other half before bed, and of course throughout the day too. It's a very big task. I also drink as much water as I do because sometimes when you think you're hungry, you're actually dehydrated. And I believe that if you're not drinking enough water, you increase your chances of pulled muscles, aches, and fatigue.

FULL NAME: Bryce Aron Max Harper

HEIGHT/WEIGHT: 6'3", 220 lbs

BORN: October 16, 1992, in Las Vegas, NV

POSITION: Outfielder

DRAFT: Drafted by the Washington Nationals in the 1st round (1st) of the 2010 MLB Draft

HIGH SCHOOL: Las Vegas High School (Las Vegas, NV)

COLLEGE: College of Southern Nevada (Henderson, NV)

AWARDS AND RECOGNITION: 6x NL All-Star; 2018 NL Home Run Derby Champion; 2012 NL ROY; 2015 NL MVP; 2015 NL Silver Slugger Award; 2015 NL Hank Aaron Award; 2015 NL home run leader

My go-to drink after a tough workout is coconut water infused with pineapple juice. I love raw pressed juices of all kinds, especially with kale and celery. I'm a big kale person. I love watermelon juice too. For a protein drink, I really enjoy almond milk with cinnamon and honey. I add cayenne to it also—cayenne just flushes out your whole system, and I enjoy the taste of it. I'll also fill a jug with water and add cucumber with a little mint. I'll drink that throughout the day just to detox. Keep it goin', keep it flowin'.

When I go to Florida for Spring Training, I buy honey fresh from a local farm and eat a scoop of it every day to alleviate my allergies. I'd rather do this than take medicine. Some may think I'm crazy, but it works for me. And honey is always my favorite natural sweetener.

I try to eat the rainbow of vegetables like purple or red cabbage, squash,

> *"I went gluten-free because it just made me feel better and healthier. I was cautious about it when I started, but the longer I went without gluten, the better I felt. The biggest difference is my energy level, which is through the roof. I feel great every day."*

kale, spinach, and zucchini. Each vegetable has a different health benefit, so I try to mix it up every day. And I can't live without mango. I eat mango with a little bit of pepper on it. I love that!

My pre-batting practice lunch is usually sautéed kale with a little protein and a sweet potato. And for a pregame snack I'll have a slice of gluten-free bread with peanut butter and honey on top or a smashed avocado with salt and pepper. It gives me good energy.

Dinner always includes a protein or a carb like gluten-free pasta. I try to stay away from chicken unless it's the middle of the day. I don't know why I don't enjoy chicken at night—unless it's in pasta or salad or something like that. I love Italian food. A good Bolognese or a mushroom sauce over gluten-free pasta is delicious.

Besides eating smart, I also do yoga twice a week in the off-season. My meditation is when I'm on a baseball field in between the lines. I have distractions in my everyday life, but when I get on the field, nothing else can get to me. When I am out there I am ready to be on the field, and I enjoy what I do.

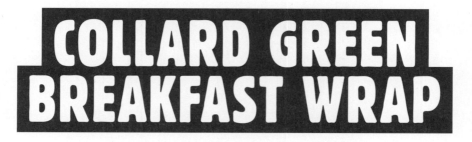

COLLARD GREEN BREAKFAST WRAP

SERVES: *1* // **PREP:** *15 minutes* // **COOK:** *5 minutes*

For a new spin on a classic wrap, try collard greens instead of the traditional tortillas and other carb-filled wraps. Dark leafy greens like collards are an excellent calcium source for breakfast or lunch wraps. Choose more flavorful dark meat chicken instead of the usual white meat, and add a touch of aromatic smoked salt.

1 large whole collard leaf

1½ teaspoons coconut oil

4 ounces ground dark meat chicken

1 large egg

1 small garlic clove, grated

2 tablespoons chopped fresh cilantro

⅛ teaspoon smoked salt

Freshly ground pepper

¼ avocado, chopped

1 cup loosely packed baby arugula, chopped

1 lime wedge

1. Remove the bottom portion of the collard stem. Use the back of a spoon to flatten out the remaining part of the stem.

2. In a medium saucepan fitted with a steamer basket, bring 2 inches of water to a boil. Place the leaf in the basket, cover, and steam for 2 to 3 minutes, until softened just enough to be pliable. Remove from the basket and lay on a flat surface while you make the filling.

3. In a medium nonstick skillet over medium-high heat, heat the oil. Add the chicken and cook, breaking it up with a wooden spoon, for about 2 minutes, until no pink remains and the meat is cooked through.

4. Crack the egg into the skillet and stir with a wooden spoon until the egg is cooked to your liking, about 30 seconds. Off the heat, stir in the garlic, cilantro, and smoked salt. Season with pepper to taste.

5. Spoon the avocado on top of the steamed leaf and top evenly with the arugula. Mound the chicken-egg mixture in the middle. Fold in the edges of the leaf and roll it up tightly (like a burrito). Cut in half crosswise. Serve with a lime wedge.

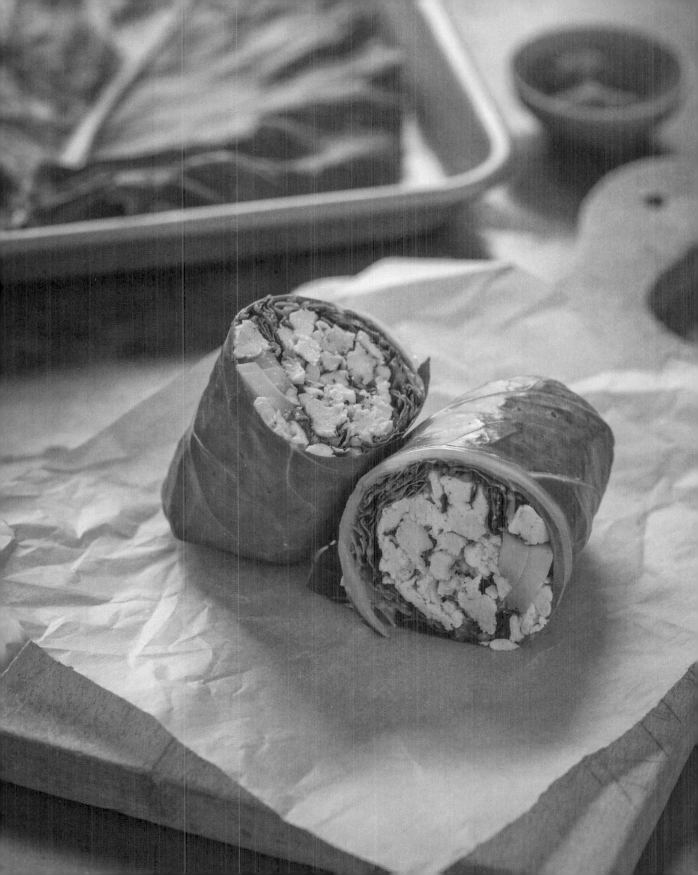

QUINOA LOAF

with Roasted Red Cabbage

SERVES: *4 to 6* // **PREP:** *30 minutes* // **COOK:** *1 hour 5 minutes*

When it comes to eating vegetables, follow Bryce Harper's lead and eat a rainbow of colors. This protein-packed quinoa loaf with a medley of veggies gets the job done.

1 medium sweet potato

1 tablespoon coconut oil, plus more for the pan

¾ cup diced carrots

¾ cup diced celery

½ cup diced bell pepper

½ cup diced shallots

3 cups cooked white quinoa (see page 13)

¼ cup brown rice flour

2 tablespoons ground flaxseeds

½ cup sliced almonds

2 large eggs, lightly beaten

½ teaspoon cider vinegar

2 tablespoons chopped fresh herbs, any combination of rosemary, flat-leaf parsley, and/or thyme

Salt and freshly ground pepper

2 tablespoons extra-virgin olive oil (optional)

Roasted Red Cabbage (recipe follows)

1. Preheat the oven to 375°F.

2. Bake the sweet potato on a baking sheet for 30 to 35 minutes, until it just starts to get soft.

Let sit until cool enough to handle, then dice the potato into small pieces for a total of 1 cup.

3. Raise the oven temperature to 400°F. Coat a 1½-quart rectangular baking dish with coconut oil.

4. In a large skillet, heat 1 tablespoon coconut oil over medium heat. Add the carrots, celery, bell pepper, and shallots and cook, stirring, until just softened, 5 to 6 minutes. Set aside to cool slightly.

5. In food processor, combine the quinoa, brown rice flour, and flaxseeds with ¼ cup water and pulse until the mixture resembles cookie dough, about 40 pulses. Transfer to a large bowl.

6. Add the cooked vegetables, sliced almonds, eggs, vinegar, and herbs to the quinoa mixture. Season with salt and pepper to taste. Gently fold in the sweet potato. Spread the mixture in the prepared pan, using a rubber spatula to smooth the surface.

7. Bake for 35 to 40 minutes, until the top is golden brown and the loaf feels firm when pressed in the center. If desired, drizzle olive oil over the hot loaf. Let cool for 20 minutes before cutting. Serve with roasted red cabbage.

ROASTED RED CABBAGE

SERVES: *4* // **PREP:** *10 minutes* //
COOK: *10 minutes*

6 cups thinly sliced red cabbage

2 teaspoons coconut oil, melted

1 large garlic clove, grated

2 teaspoons fresh lemon juice

Salt and freshly ground pepper

1. Preheat the oven to 450°F.

2. In a large bowl, combine the cabbage and
oil, tossing evenly to lightly coat. Divide the
cabbage between 2 baking sheets, spreading it
in an even layer. Set the bowl aside.

3. Roast the cabbage for 6 to 8 minutes,
until tender-crisp. Return the cabbage to the
bowl and toss with the garlic and lemon juice.
Season with salt and pepper to taste.

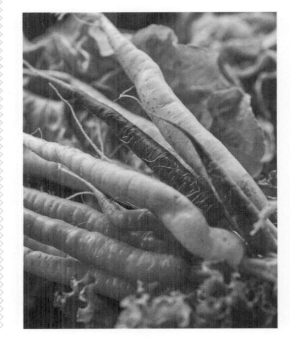

The Lineup and Game-Changing Recipes

BEEF BOLOGNESE

with Roasted Collard Greens

SERVES: 2 // **PREP:** *15 minutes* // **COOK:** *55 minutes*

Chicken livers are the secret to making an All-Star Bolognese. Just the right amount brings this classic sauce over the top. And when choosing canned tomatoes, look for organic San Marzanos; they are best for their sweetness and low acidity.

2 cups canned plum tomatoes, drained, reserving ¼ cup juice

¼ cup chicken livers

1½ teaspoons coconut oil

¼ cup chopped yellow onion

1 tablespoon minced garlic

1 tablespoon finely chopped carrot

8 ounces 85% lean grass-fed ground beef

Pinch of crushed red pepper flakes

Pinch of coconut sugar

Handful of basil leaves, torn

Salt and freshly ground pepper

6 ounces uncooked gluten-free pasta, such as spaghetti

Roasted Collard Greens (recipe follows)

1. In a blender, puree the tomatoes and chicken livers until smooth.

2. In a medium saucepan, heat the oil over medium heat. Add the onion, garlic, and carrot and cook, stirring frequently, for about 2 minutes, until the onion is golden brown. Add the beef and cook, breaking it up with a wooden spoon, for about 4 minutes, until it is cooked through and no pink remains. Add the pureed tomato mixture, the reserved tomato juice, red pepper flakes, and sugar.

3. Reduce the heat to low and simmer, stirring occasionally, especially toward the end of cooking, until thickened, about 45 minutes. Remove from the heat, fold in the basil, and season with salt and pepper to taste.

4. Bring a large pot of water to a boil. Add the pasta and cook until al dente according to the package instructions. Drain well and divide between 2 bowls. Top with the Bolognese sauce and roasted collard greens.

ROASTED COLLARD GREENS

SERVES 2 // **PREP:** *10 minutes* // **COOK:** *5 minutes*

4 cups lightly packed sliced collard greens, tough ribs removed before slicing

1½ teaspoons fresh lemon juice (optional)

Salt and freshly ground pepper

Preheat the oven to 450°F. Lay the collards on a large baking sheet and roast, stirring once, for 4 to 6 minutes, until dried and slightly crisp. Transfer to a bowl and toss with the lemon juice (if using) and salt and pepper to taste.

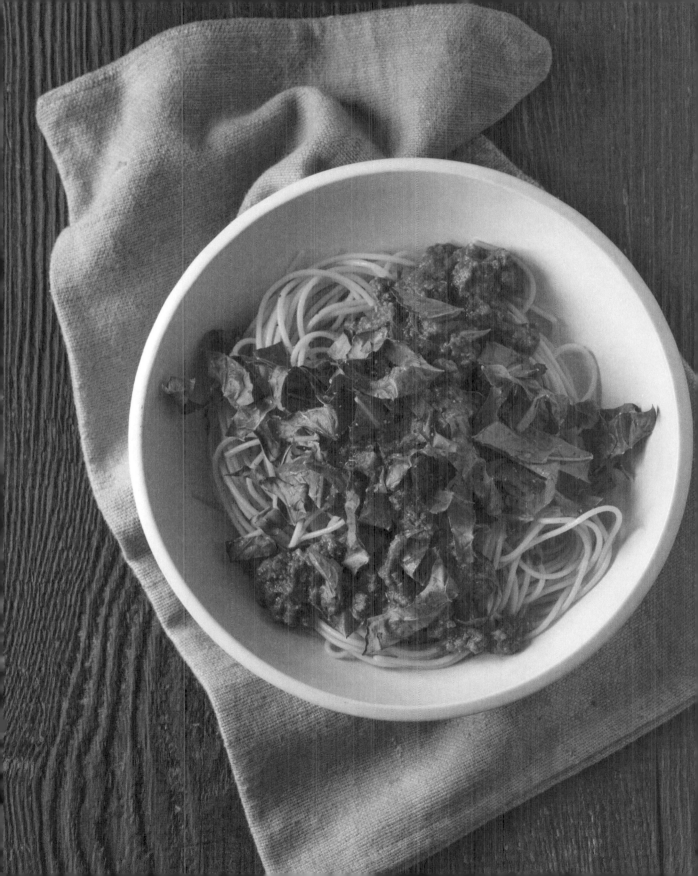

CUCUMBER MINT WATER

SERVES: *1* // **PREP:** *5 minutes*

Stay hydrated with thirst-quenching, cucumber-infused water. It's not only refreshing but also fun to make. Proper hydration helps to prevent muscle cramps, rid your body of toxins, and boost recovery.

2 cups water

4 (¼-inch-thick) cucumber slices

6 mint leaves, crushed (see Note)

Note: To muddle mint, place the mint leaves in a heavy-bottomed glass and with the flat end of a muddler gently press down and twist four or five times to release the flavor. If you do not have a muddler, you can use the back of a wooden spoon or the end of a French rolling pin.

Combine the water, cucumber, and mint in a pitcher or jar and infuse in the refrigerator overnight. Strain into glasses to serve.

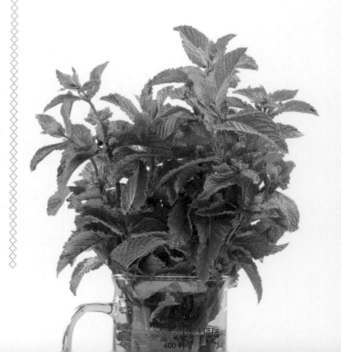

COCONUT PINEAPPLE WATER

SERVES: *1* // **PREP:** *5 minutes*

This smooth and frothy drink is full of sparkle and mouthwatering flavor. Pineapple is packed with the enzyme bromelain, which helps to reduce inflammation. When choosing coconut water, look for the organic brands found in the refrigerated section of your grocery store.

1½ cups chilled coconut water
1 cup chopped peeled pineapple
Juice and grated zest of 1 lime

In a high-powered blender, combine the coconut water, pineapple, lime juice, and zest and process for 30 seconds.

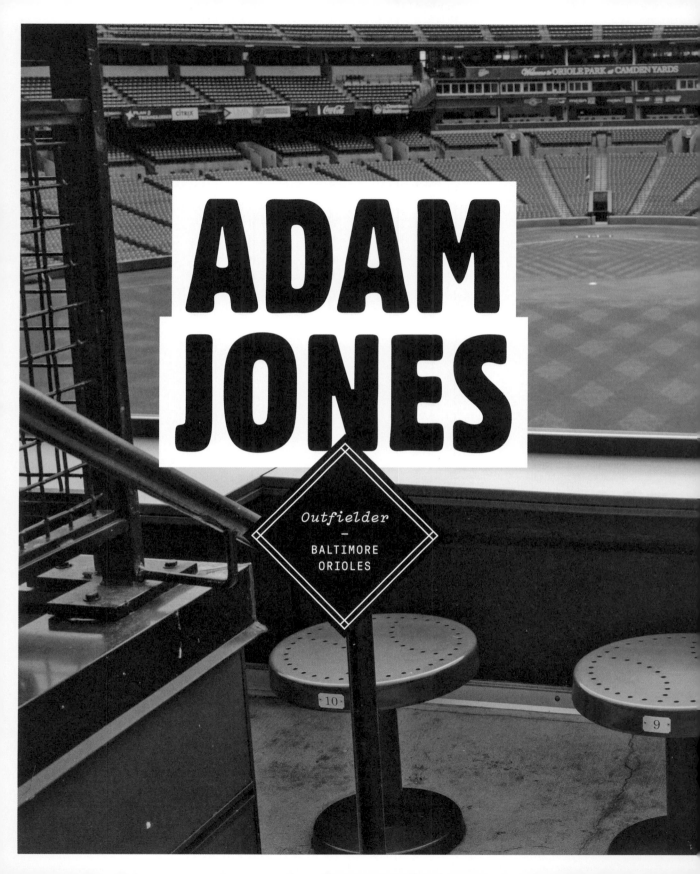

ADAM JONES

Outfielder
—
BALTIMORE ORIOLES

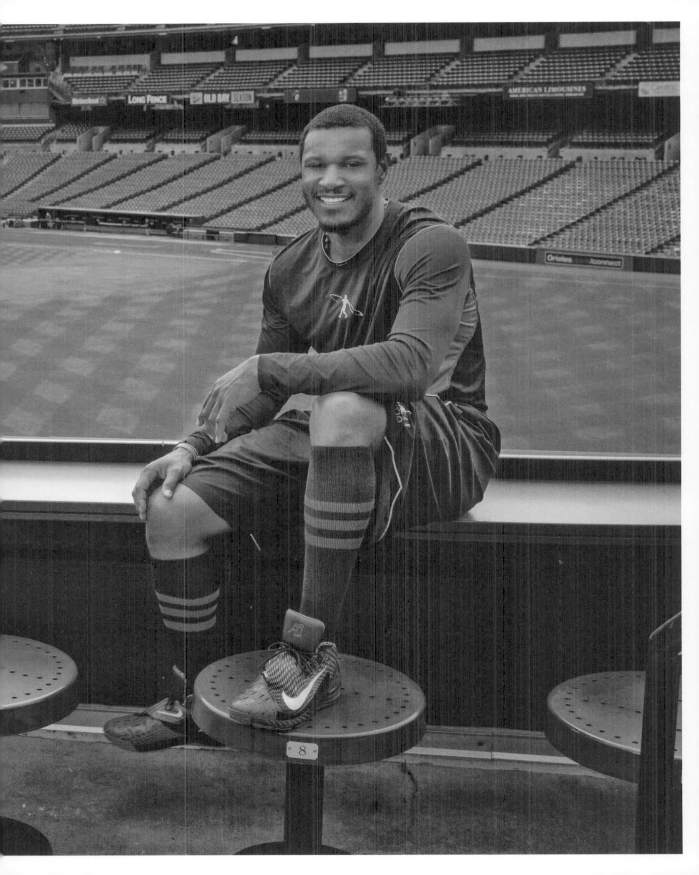

I've gained an awareness of healthy food over the last few years and I try to eat well as often as possible. I don't need to eat fried foods all the time, and I don't need to drink soda. I've really cut back on trans fats and sugar. I still eat the foods that I like, but a healthier form of them. Now I feel better after eating. I don't feel like I want to go to sleep.

For breakfast I always have an omelet with broccoli, diced jalapeños, and a little bit of cheese—it's my Spring Training go-to. During the regular season, I add oatmeal to that; I wake up at 9:00 a.m. to eat and then go back to bed, and the oatmeal helps me to sleep. I get up for the day at eleven or noon. I want to be on a schedule where I don't skip breakfast. I'd rather get it in me and go back to sleep.

I like a green juice that is light and simple. It is filled with a lot of nutrients and won't leave me feeling overloaded.

Every day I eat homemade gluten-free snacks that are similar to cookies, made with sweet potatoes and peanut butter, but no flour. I'm not gluten-free, but I try to avoid it. Our team chef, Jenny, makes me gluten-free snacks because snacks are my danger zone. She found a way to make cookies healthier for me. There

FULL NAME: Adam LaMarque Jones

HEIGHT/WEIGHT: 6'2", 215 lbs

BORN: August 1, 1985, in San Diego, CA

POSITION: Centerfielder

DRAFT: Drafted by the Seattle Mariners in the 1st round (37th) of the 2003 MLB Draft

HIGH SCHOOL: Samuel F. B. Morse High School (San Diego, CA)

AWARDS AND RECOGNITION: 5x AL All-Star; 4x AL Gold Glove Award; 2013 AL Silver Slugger Award

are no sugars or grains in them, and I feel better after eating them. I've started my son on this same path. I try to create early awareness about eating well. As an athlete, I try to eat foods that reduce inflammation in my joints and my muscles because I need to play every day.

My favorite smoothie is one I call the "kitchen sink." It basically includes every vegetable and every fruit I can find—spinach, blueberries, strawberries, mango, beet juice, and carrots plus peanut butter and honey—all in one smoothie. I'm not a big milk drinker. I'll drink almond milk, but I prefer water.

I'm a fan of "superfoods" like spirulina and turmeric. I drink a shot of turmeric in the morning. It gets me going. And I drink wheatgrass shots. There's a set-up in our clubhouse kitchen to make them.

Usually I'm really hungry after working out in the afternoon and I'll eat chili, which satisfies me immediately. Then I still have enough time to develop an appetite for dinner. I like grass-fed bison and venison. I notice now that if I eat my meals on time and closer together I don't overeat; instead I feel satisfied. Most of my teammates are

"*I'm a fan of 'superfoods' like spirulina and turmeric. I drink a shot of turmeric in the morning. It gets me going. And I drink wheatgrass shots. There's a set-up in our clubhouse kitchen to make them.*"

on board too. No one goes to fast-food places anymore, and if they do it's the exception. It's not just having someone cook for you; it's the awareness of what is good for you. It's knowing what your body likes and doesn't like.

Dinner always includes kale—it's a focal point. Kale is one of the foods I didn't like when I first started eating well. I learned to massage it with some lemon and a little salt and pepper to make it taste better. There's always some sort of salad with dinner. And I didn't like beets, but now I like them in a juice.

You can eat healthily and still enjoy the food you like—it's about finding a happy medium. I still like cheese steaks, burgers, and pizza, but now I eliminate bad dough, bad cheese, and bad tomato sauces. I eat gluten-free noodles now. The goal isn't to get away from eating these foods entirely; it's finding healthier versions of them. Get away from processed stuff. Instead of chips and salsa for a snack, have hummus and carrots.

Our lives are hectic and often we're pulled in many directions. To find peace and serenity, I try to just get out to the ocean with my wife and kids. There's nothing better.

CHICKPEA BOWL

with Jalapeño Tahini

SERVES: *2* // **PREP:** *25 minutes* // **COOK:** *20 minutes*

The high-fiber and protein-filled chickpeas are just the start of what makes this completely satisfying main meal so good, hot or cold. For a next-day cold meal, just refrigerate, but keep the tahini sauce separate until serving.

1 cup diced peeled butternut squash

½ teaspoon coconut oil, melted

2 cups tender sprigs trimmed broccoli rabe

1½ cups cooked chickpeas (see page 12)

3 tablespoons shaved red onion

2 tablespoons shredded carrot

½ teaspoon ground turmeric

½ teaspoon minced garlic

1 tablespoon extra-virgin olive oil

Salt and freshly ground pepper

Jalapeño Tahini (recipe follows)

1. Preheat the oven to 400°F.

2. Toss the butternut squash with the coconut oil and spread on a baking sheet in a single layer. Roast for 15 to 20 minutes, stirring occasionally, until golden and cooked through.

3. In a saucepan fitted with a steamer basket, bring 1 inch of water to a boil. Add the broccoli rabe, cover, and steam until tender, 1 to

1½ minutes. When cool enough to handle, coarsely chop and transfer to a large bowl.

4. Add the roasted squash, chickpeas, red onion, carrot, turmeric, garlic, and olive oil to the bowl with the rabe and toss to combine. Season with salt and pepper to taste. Divide between 2 bowls and top with 1 to 2 tablespoons jalapeño tahini.

JALAPEÑO TAHINI

SERVES: *2* // **PREP:** *5 minutes*

2 tablespoons tahini (be sure to stir it well first)

1½ teaspoons minced seeded jalapeño

1½ tablespoons fresh lemon juice

Salt

In a small bowl, whisk together the tahini, 1 tablespoon water (or more if you want a thinner sauce), jalapeño, and lemon juice. Season with salt to taste.

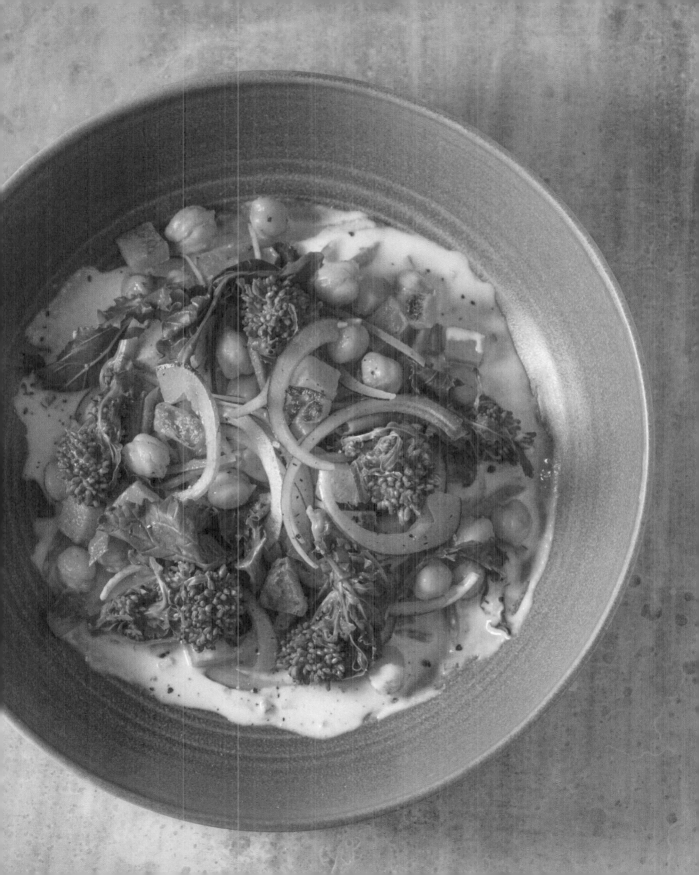

BISON CHILI

SERVES: 4 // **PREP:** 20 minutes // **COOK:** 40 minutes

A bowl of nourishing chili is Adam Jones's preference after a tough workout. The richness of the tomatoes and just the right mix of peppers hit it out of the park. For a lean meat alternative to bison, venison works well.

1 tablespoon coconut oil

¼ cup finely chopped yellow onion

1 tablespoon minced garlic

6 ounces ground bison

½ teaspoon ground cumin

½ teaspoon chili powder

⅛ teaspoon cayenne (optional)

1½ cups finely chopped bell pepper

⅓ cup finely chopped poblano pepper

1½ cups tomato puree

Salt and freshly ground pepper

2 cups thinly sliced collard greens, tough ribs removed first

1 tablespoon fresh lemon juice

1½ teaspoons extra-virgin olive oil

1. In a large saucepan, heat the coconut oil over medium heat. Add the onion and garlic and cook, stirring frequently, until softened, 1 to 2 minutes. Add the bison. Cook, stirring and breaking up the meat with a wooden spoon, until cooked through and no pink remains, 3 to 4 minutes. Add the cumin, chili powder, and cayenne, if using, and cook, stirring, for 30 seconds.

2. Add the bell and poblano peppers, tomato puree, and ½ cup water. Reduce the heat to medium-low and cook, stirring occasionally (especially toward the end of cooking), until thickened, about 35 minutes. Season with salt and pepper to taste.

3. Place the collards in a medium bowl and use your hands to massage the leaves with the lemon juice and olive oil. Season with salt and pepper to taste. Divide the chili between 2 bowls and top with the collard greens.

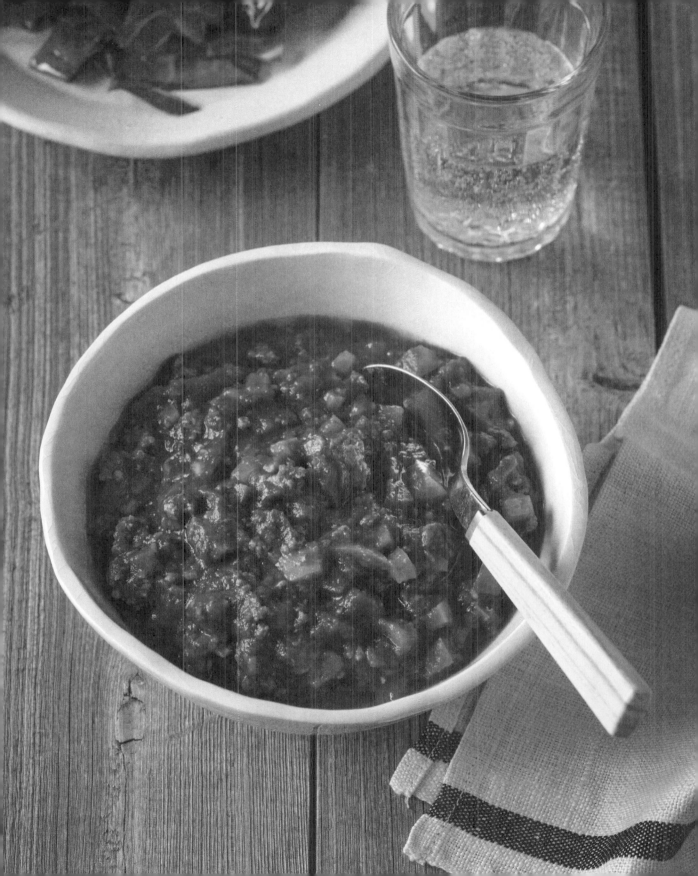

CINNAMON MACAROONS

MAKES: *about ten 2-inch cookies* // **PREP:** *15 minutes* // **COOK:** *1 hour 5 minutes*

The sweet potato is the secret ingredient in these guilt-free snacks inspired by Adam Jones. Crunchy on the outside and creamy in the middle, they are heavenly when eaten warm, straight out of the oven.

1 small sweet potato (or ¼ cup leftover mashed baked sweet potato)

3 tablespoons almond or walnut butter

2 tablespoons pure maple syrup

2 tablespoons almond flour

1 teaspoon ground cinnamon

Pinch of salt

1. Preheat the oven to 375°F.

2. Place the sweet potato on a baking sheet and bake for 40 to 45 minutes, until soft. Set aside until cool enough to handle, then remove the skin and mash until smooth. Measure out ¼ cup and reserve the rest for another use.

3. If you cooked the sweet potato in advance, preheat the oven to 375°F. Line a baking sheet with a nonstick silicone mat.

4. In a medium bowl, mash the sweet potato and almond butter together with a fork until combined. Add the maple syrup, flour, cinnamon, and salt and mix well. Using a tablespoon, drop walnut-size rounds of batter onto the prepared baking sheet, spacing them 2 inches apart.

5. Bake for 12 minutes. Using an offset spatula, flip the macaroons and press gently so they don't tip over. Bake for an additional 7 to 9 minutes, until slightly crispy on top, with browned edges. Let cool for 5 minutes on the baking sheet. Cookies are best eaten when freshly baked and warm, but they will keep in an airtight container in the refrigetator for up to 2 days.

KITCHEN SINK SMOOTHIE

SERVES: 1 // **PREP:** 15 minutes // **COOK:** 45 minutes

This creative take on Adam Jones's aptly named smoothie (pictured on page 69) is insanely good. Loaded with protein, it's also an easy way to add more fruits and vegetables to your diet. Enjoy as a satisfying drink or a post-workout snack.

1 small sweet potato (or ½ cup leftover mashed baked sweet potato)

½ cup quartered hulled strawberries

⅔ cup chilled almond milk

1½ teaspoons almond butter

2 tablespoons pomegranate seeds

½ teaspoon spirulina (optional)

1 tablespoon rolled oats (optional)

Handful of spinach (optional)

Whatever else you can find that will blend (e.g., leftover cooked quinoa or brown rice, massaged kale, blueberries, raspberries, etc.)

1. Preheat the oven to 375°F.

2. Place the sweet potato on a baking sheet and bake until soft, 40 to 45 minutes. When cool enough to handle, remove the skin and mash some of the potato until you have ½ cup. Save the rest for your next smoothie or cinnamon macaroons (see opposite).

3. In a high-powered blender, combine all the ingredients until smooth.

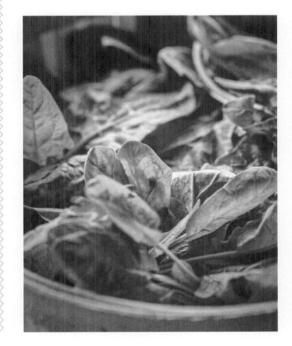

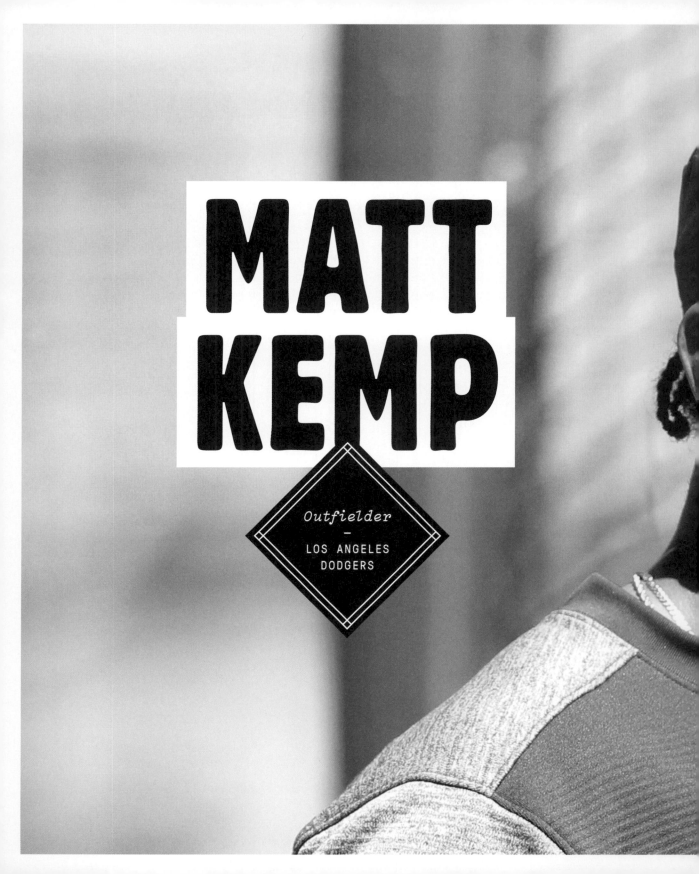

MATT KEMP

Outfielder
–
LOS ANGELES DODGERS

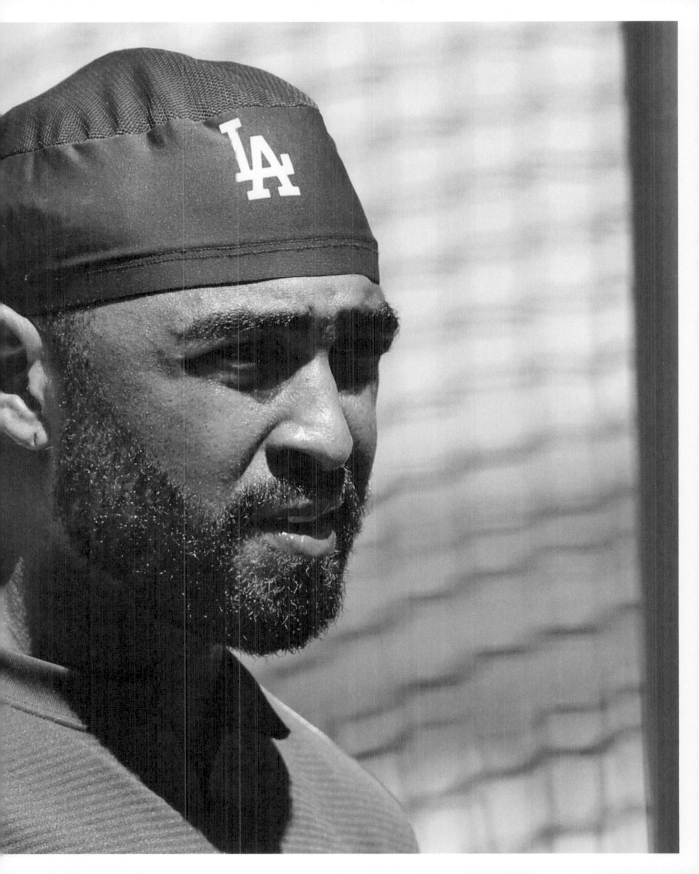

Recently in the off-season, I changed my eating habits. The main reason was because I wanted to be faster and play the outfield better in order to compete with our crowded competition.

One of the biggest changes to my diet was to eat six small meals a day, and mostly protein. Playing in LA is great when it comes to eating all of the healthy stuff.

You can make all kinds of things for breakfast. I have oatmeal for breakfast, but you can make your own healthy choices like nutritious wraps with protein and vegetables, or if you want something lighter, a protein shake is always good too.

I eliminated dairy from my diet because it doesn't sit right in my stomach. Dairy is tough for me to digest. I've heard that milk affects a lot of people the same way.

When I'm hungry and looking for a snack, I like homemade granola bars with nuts in them for protein and healthy fat. Protein bars don't need a lot of ingredients to be good, and when they are homemade, you know they are filled with the healthy stuff.

FULL NAME: Matthew Ryan Kemp

HEIGHT/WEIGHT: 6'4", 210 lbs

BORN: September 23, 1984, in Midwest City, OK

POSITION: Outfielder

DRAFT: Drafted by the Los Angeles Dodgers in the 6th round of the 2003 MLB Draft

HIGH SCHOOL: Midwest City High School (Midwest City, OK)

AWARDS AND RECOGNITION: 3x NL All-Star; 2x NL Gold Glove Award; 2x NL Silver Slugger Award; 2011 NL Hank Aaron Award; 2011 NL home run leader; 2011 NL RBI leader; hit for the cycle on August 14, 2015

Sometimes it is easier to drink my veggies. When our team is on the road, fresh juices are a convenient and healthy option when I am not eating enough green vegetables. When I am home, I like to make fresh green juices with a bit of lemon. I don't put any other fruit in them because I don't eat a lot of fruit in general.

I've cut back on eating carbs at night. I don't eat them after seven o'clock. My meals are primarily protein like salmon, chicken, and lean meat. For dinner, I eat protein without the carbs and a green vegetable. I don't feel bloated after eating this way and it helps me to sleep better.

I like almost all vegetables, including the popular kale. I eat most of the good stuff. It is pointless to work out and then eat poorly. Eating a burger right after your workout defeats the purpose. And if you're trying to lose weight, that's not the right approach.

It is fun to come up with new ways of eating smart because in the end I like the way I feel afterward. But sometimes healthy eating is all about just eating for fuel. If I am working out and doing a lot, I will eat more because my body is telling me,

"I've cut back on eating carbs at night. I don't eat them after seven o'clock. My meals are primarily protein like salmon, chicken, and lean meat. For dinner, I eat protein without the carbs and a green vegetable. I don't feel bloated after eating this way and it helps me to sleep better."

"Dude, you're hungry and if you don't eat, you're going to pass out." I know to listen to what my body needs.

When I eat poorly, I am super moody.
I've learned that you are what you eat, because I know when I eat well it affects me physically and mentally. Not only do I feel great, but my mind is clear and I can think straight. In the end, I know I am much more productive.

BISON MEATBALLS

with Cauliflower Rice and Spicy Spinach

SERVES: *4* // **PREP:** *15 minutes* // **COOK:** *10 minutes*

As an excellent source of lean protein, bison has become a favorite among many players. Cauliflower rice is the perfect noncarb choice to accompany the meatballs. For some tasty greens, spicy spinach is just right.

2½ tablespoons coconut oil

2 tablespoons minced seeded serrano pepper

1½ tablespoons minced garlic

1 pound ground bison

1 large egg

2 tablespoons almond flour

½ teaspoon smoked paprika

½ teaspoon salt

Cauliflower Rice (recipe follows)

Spicy Spinach (recipe follows)

1. In a small skillet, heat ½ tablespoon of the oil over medium heat. Add the serrano and garlic and cook, stirring, until golden brown, about 2 minutes. Transfer to a large bowl and add the bison, egg, flour, paprika, and salt.

2. Using your hands, mix all ingredients until evenly combined. Use a #60 scoop (about 1 tablespoon) to portion the meatballs and roll them in your hands to shape. You should have about thirty-six 1-inch meatballs.

3. In a large skillet, heat 1 tablespoon of the oil over medium heat. Add half of the meatballs and cook, turning often, until golden brown and cooked through, 4 to 5 minutes total. Transfer to a plate and cover to keep warm. Repeat with the remaining 1 tablespoon oil and meatballs.

4. Serve with cauliflower rice and spicy spinach.

CAULIFLOWER RICE

SERVES: *4* // **PREP:** *15 minutes* //
COOK: *5 minutes*

6 cups chopped cauliflower florets
2 tablespoons coconut oil
¾ cup finely chopped yellow onion
½ cup chopped fresh flat-leaf parsley
Salt and freshly ground pepper

1. In a food processor, pulse the cauliflower for 15 to 20 seconds until it resembles grains of rice (once processed, you'll have about 3¾ cups).

2. In a large skillet, heat the oil over medium heat. Add the onion and cook, stirring, until golden brown, about 3 minutes.

3. Add the cauliflower to the skillet and cook, stirring, until softened, 2 to 3 minutes. Remove from the heat and fold in the parsley. Season with salt and pepper to taste.

SPICY SPINACH

SERVES: *4* // **PREP:** *5 minutes* //
COOK: *5 minutes*

2 pounds baby spinach
1 tablespoon coconut oil
2 tablespoons minced garlic
¼ teaspoon cayenne
2 tablespoons fresh lemon juice (optional)
Salt and freshly ground pepper

1. In a 5- to 6-quart pot with a steamer basket, bring 1 inch of water to a boil. Add half the spinach, cover, and steam until slightly wilted, about 5 seconds. Uncover and stir in the remaining spinach. Cover and steam until just wilted, 15 to 20 seconds. Remove the steamer basket and let the spinach cool enough to handle. Squeeze some of the water from the spinach, place in a medium bowl, and cover to keep warm.

2. In a small skillet, heat the oil over medium heat. Add the garlic and cook until golden brown, about 2 minutes. Add the garlic, cayenne, and lemon juice (if using) to the spinach. Season with salt and pepper to taste and stir to combine.

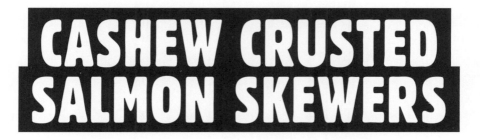

CASHEW CRUSTED SALMON SKEWERS

SERVES: 2 // **PREP:** 5 minutes // **COOK:** 10 minutes

These salmon skewers are super satisfying for entertaining hungry guests, a light lunch, or a sensational snack. The crispy sesame seed coating is the impeccable complement to the tender salmon. Each morsel is bursting with flavor and texture.

8 ounces skinned salmon fillets, pin bones removed

½ cup ground raw cashews

2 tablespoons raw sesame seeds, white or black

¼ teaspoon salt plus more to taste

1 tablespoon tahini

2 teaspoons fresh lemon juice

6 (4-inch) bamboo wooden skewers

1½ tablespoons coconut oil, melted

1½ teaspoons sesame oil

1 tablespoon sliced scallions, white and green parts

2 lemon wedges, for serving

1. Cut the salmon into 6 equal pieces. Mix the cashews, sesame seeds, and ¼ teaspoon salt in a shallow, wide bowl.

2. In another small bowl, whisk together 1½ tablespoons water, tahini, and lemon juice. Season with salt.

3. Toss the salmon in the tahini mixture until evenly coated. Dredge the salmon in the nut mixture to coat evenly.

4. In a medium nonstick skillet, heat the oil over medium heat until hot but not smoking. Cook the salmon, turning, until golden brown on all sides, about 8 minutes total. Remove from the pan and cool slightly.

5. Skewer each salmon piece securely (so it resembles a lollipop). Sprinkle with scallions, drizzle with sesame oil, and serve with lemon wedges.

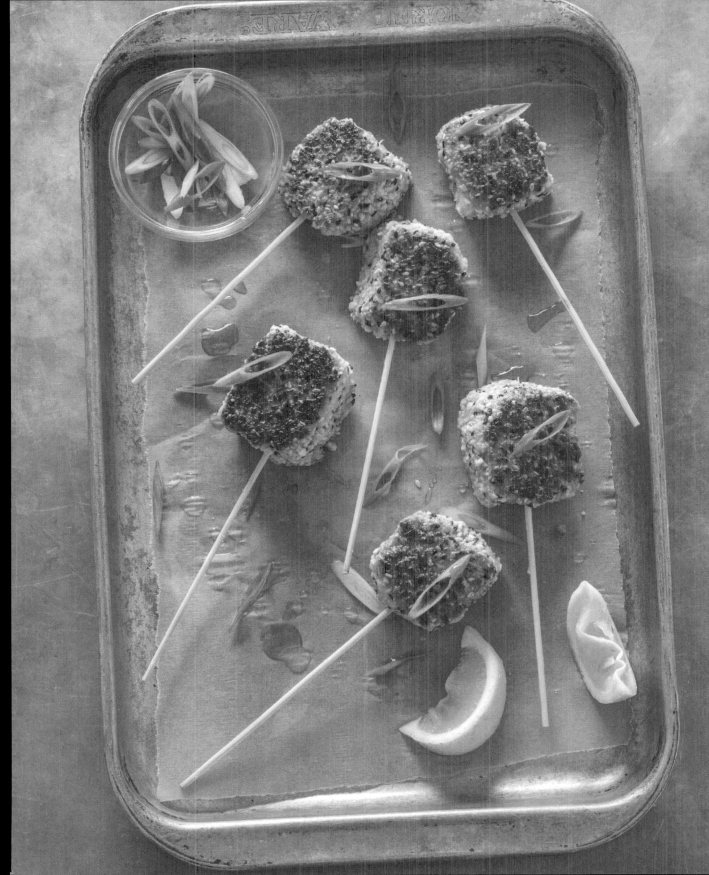

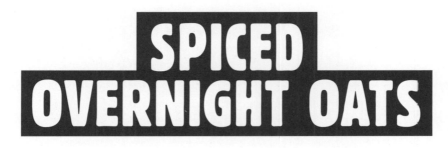

SPICED OVERNIGHT OATS

SERVES: *2* // **PREP:** *5 minutes, plus soaking time* // **COOK:** *5 minutes*

Protein-rich oatmeal is a favorite breakfast for Matt Kemp. Cooking in almond milk adds a creamy texture without the dairy. When pressed for time, the oats can be prepared overnight so they're ready to go the next morning. Added toppings are optional, so spice it up or simply choose whichever appeals to you.

1 cup gluten-free steel-cut oats

½ cup unsweetened almond milk (see page 13)

½ teaspoon ground cinnamon

¼ teaspoon ground nutmeg

¼ teaspoon ground allspice

2 teaspoons maple syrup (optional)

Pinch of salt

½ cup sliced banana or fresh berries (optional)

2 tablespoons nuts and seeds (optional)

1. The night before, in a medium saucepan over medium heat, bring 3 cups water and the oats to a boil and cook for 1 minute. Remove from the heat, cover, and refrigerate overnight in the saucepan.

2. In the morning, the oats will have soaked up the water and softened to a perfect consistency. Add the almond milk, spices, maple syrup (if using), and salt to the oats. Heat over medium-low heat until hot, stirring occasionally, about 4 minutes. Top with fresh fruit, nuts, and seeds, if desired.

WARM SWEET POTATO KALE BOWL

SERVES: *2* // **PREP:** *20 minutes* // **COOK:** *30 minutes*

Kale is king for this bowl of nourishing comfort food. With the added sweet potato and rice, there are plenty of hearty ingredients to make this a substantial meal for lunch, dinner, or even breakfast.

2 cups diced peeled sweet potato

½ teaspoon coconut oil, melted

3 cups chopped curly kale leaves, tough stems removed first

1½ tablespoons fresh lime juice

1½ tablespoons fresh lemon juice

Salt and freshly ground pepper

2 cups cooked basmati or jasmine rice, warm (see page 13)

2 tablespoons thinly sliced scallions, white and green parts

2 tablespoons chopped fresh cilantro

1 tablespoon extra-virgin olive oil

1. Preheat the oven to 400°F.

2. Toss the sweet potato with the coconut oil and arrange in one layer on a baking sheet. Roast for about 30 minutes, until tender and golden.

3. In a saucepan fitted with a steamer basket, bring 1 inch of water to a boil. Put the kale in the basket, cover, and steam for 15 to 20 seconds. Remove from the heat and transfer to a large bowl. Toss the kale with the roasted sweet potato and lime and lemon juice. Season with salt and pepper to taste.

4. In another bowl, toss the cooked rice with the scallions, cilantro, and olive oil. Season with salt and pepper to taste. Divide the rice and sweet potato mixture between 2 bowls and serve.

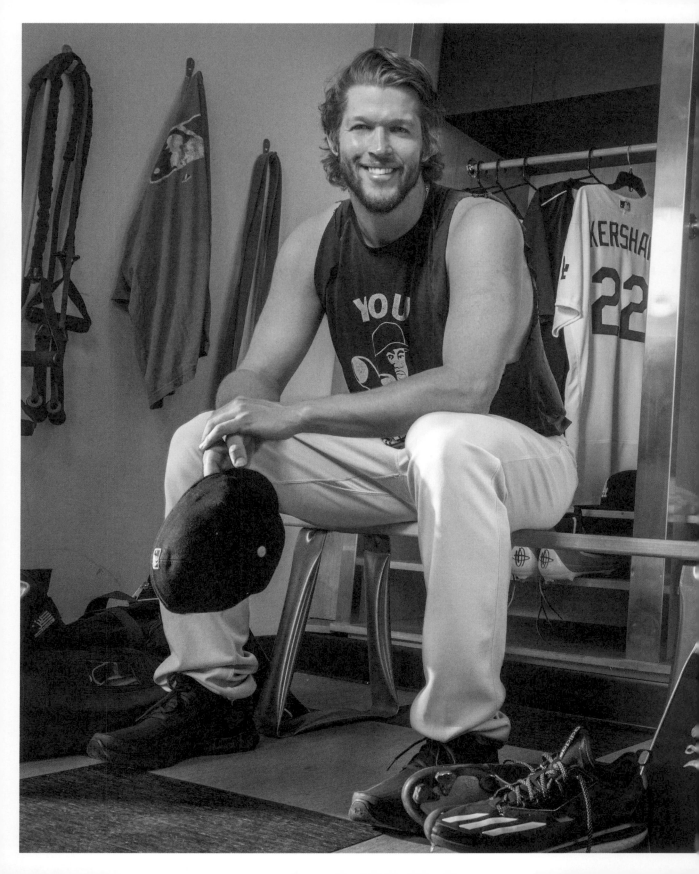

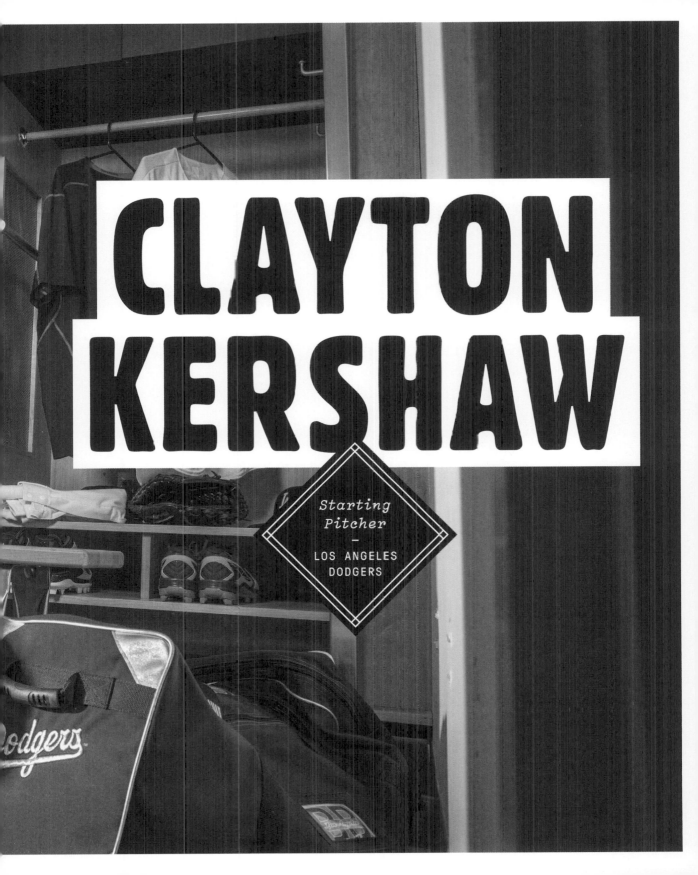

CLAYTON KERSHAW

Starting Pitcher

—

LOS ANGELES DODGERS

My motivation for eating smart began in high school, as I had always been a chubby kid. Then I started growing in high school and eating better, and it all came together for me.

My breakfast routine depends on whether I'm pitching or not—on the days I pitch, I always eat a full breakfast. On the days I don't, I'm usually a sleep-in guy and don't eat a lot—a banana and yogurt. That's it. I like to work out on an empty stomach. Then I go to the field, and I'll have a big lunch after that.

On days I don't pitch, I'll just make a healthy smoothie after our game because our games end so late, and I don't want to overeat. I'll put spinach or kale, almond milk, blueberries, strawberries, some protein powder, and cinnamon in the smoothie. After a tough workout I'll usually have a shake with protein powder and amino acids, mixed with water. I also love pineapple—can't live without it.

Our clubhouse is completely organic now—there has been a complete shift in food. For lunch I usually have a protein like grilled or broiled chicken and a complex carbohydrate like brown rice. That is my go-to lunch. And we now have grass-fed beef in our clubhouse, so I'll have that for dinner.

I recently discovered that I like salmon sushi, but I eat it without the white rice so it's healthier. I never liked it before, but since I like salmon so much I thought I'd give it a try, and now it's the only sushi I eat.

I try to have the same workout routine between each start, and that way— every fifth day—I know I've done everything I possibly can do to be ready for the game. A routine helps me with peace of mind. My biggest workout day is the one after I pitch. It's my biggest day for running and other cardio, but not a whole lot of throwing. Over the next few days, I progressively reduce my running and cardio workout and increase my throwing until the day I'm scheduled to pitch again.

Being a parent allows me to remove myself from the game a little bit, and it's really important for me to find that balance. Before I got married and had kids, the game sometimes would wear on me, especially if I pitched poorly. I would just wear it for four days. Having a family really helped me. Once I go home, I kind of turn it off.

FULL NAME: Clayton Edward Kershaw

HEIGHT/WEIGHT: 6'4", 228 lbs

BORN: March 19, 1988, in Dallas, TX

POSITION: Pitcher

DRAFT: Drafted by the Los Angeles Dodgers in the 1st round (7th) of the 2006 MLB Draft

HIGH SCHOOL: Highland Park High School (University Park, TX)

AWARDS AND RECOGNITION: 7x NL All-Star; 5x NL ERA title; 3x NL Cy Young Award; 2011 NL Pitching Triple Crown (Wins, ERA, Ks); 2014 NL MVP; 2011 NL Gold Glove Award; 2014 no-hitter; 2012 Roberto Clemente Award; 3x NL wins leader; 3x NL strikeout leader

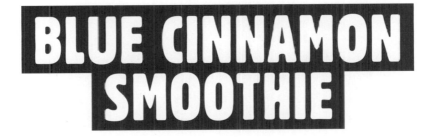

BLUE CINNAMON SMOOTHIE

SERVES: *1* // **PREP:** *5 minutes*

The combination of dates, cinnamon, and vanilla creates a light and chocolaty taste without any chocolate. Blueberries are a natural low-calorie sweetener and are full of healthy antioxidants that help minimize inflammation and improve brain health.

1½ cups chilled unsweetened almond milk (see page 13)

1 cup frozen blueberries, broken up

¼ avocado

1 pitted date

½ teaspoon ground cinnamon

⅛ teaspoon vanilla extract

In a high-powered blender, combine the milk, blueberries, avocado, date, cinnamon, and vanilla and process until smooth.

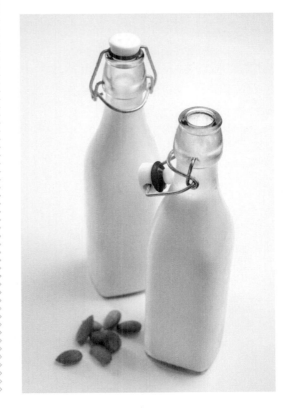

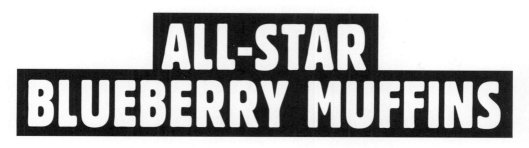

ALL-STAR BLUEBERRY MUFFINS

MAKES: *6 muffins* // **PREP:** *10 minutes* // **COOK:** *20 minutes*

Made with almond flour and oat flour, these gluten-free blueberry muffins are super satisfying without being overly filling. Whip up a batch (or two or three) for breakfast, as a treat, or as an after-school snack.

¾ **cup almond flour**

¾ **cup oat flour**

⅛ **teaspoon baking powder**

⅛ **teaspoon baking soda**

⅛ **teaspoon salt**

½ **cup frozen blueberries, broken up**

1 **large egg**

½ **cup full-fat canned coconut milk (shake well before measuring)**

3 **tablespoons maple syrup**

1½ **teaspoons coconut oil, melted**

1. Preheat the oven to 375°F. Line 6 wells of a muffin tin with paper baking cups.

2. In a medium bowl, whisk together the almond flour, oat flour, baking powder, baking soda, and salt. Mix in the blueberries until well combined.

3. In a separate bowl, whisk together the egg, milk, maple syrup, and oil. Fold the wet ingredients into the dry until evenly incorporated.

4. Fill the muffin cups evenly with batter (about ⅓ cup each) and bake for about 20 minutes, until a toothpick inserted in the center comes out clean and the top is firm to the touch.

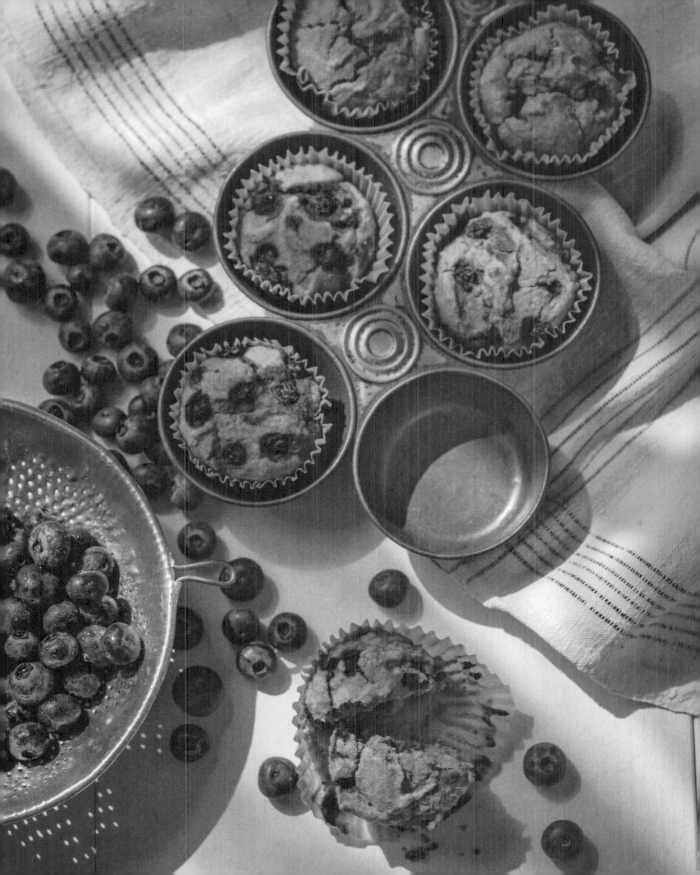

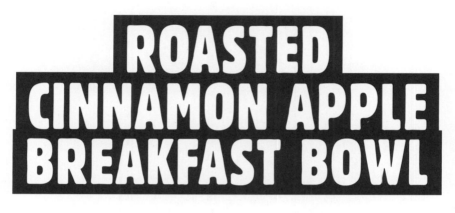

ROASTED CINNAMON APPLE BREAKFAST BOWL

SERVES: 2 // **PREP:** 5 minutes // **COOK:** 20 minutes

Instead of the usual yogurt and fruit breakfast, why not try this protein-packed quinoa bowl featuring baked cinnamon apples and banana? Quinoa is full of iron, calcium, magnesium, and fiber, all of which help boost antioxidant levels and your immune system.

1 teaspoon coconut oil, melted

½ teaspoon ground cinnamon

1 medium apple (such as Fuji), cored and cut into ½-inch slices

2 cups cooked white quinoa, warm (see page 13)

½ cup unsweetened almond milk (see page 13)

2 teaspoons maple syrup (optional)

1 ripe medium banana, sliced

1 tablespoon hemp hearts

1 tablespoon pumpkin seeds

1. Preheat the oven to 400°F.

2. In a small bowl, combine the oil and cinnamon. Toss the apple slices in the mixture and arrange on a baking sheet. Bake until softened, 18 to 20 minutes. Set the apple aside to cool slightly, then chop coarsely.

3. Divide the quinoa between 2 bowls and pour ¼ cup milk into each bowl. Drizzle maple syrup over the quinoa if you'd like.

4. Divide the banana and apple between the 2 bowls and sprinkle the hemp hearts and pumpkin seeds over top. Serve immediately.

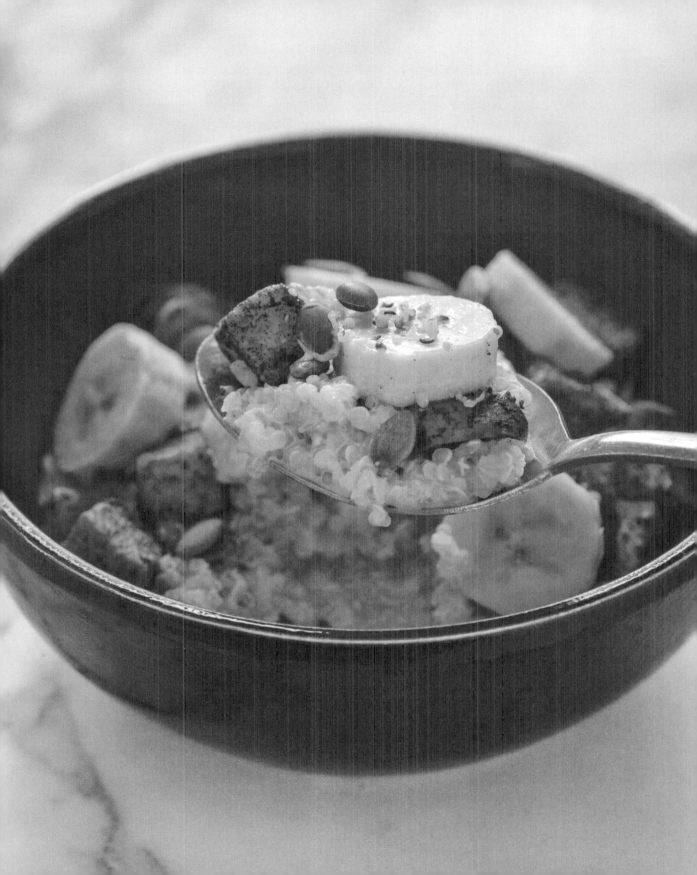

SALMON NORI ROLL

SERVES: *2* // **PREP:** *30 minutes* // **COOK:** *15 minutes*

This wrap is full of crunchy vegetables and tangy flavors, all rolled up in the Japanese seaweed known as nori. Creamy avocado is key to holding it all together. Enjoy these rolls right away while the nori is still crisp.

½ teaspoon coconut oil, melted

6 ounces wild salmon fillets, pin bones removed

Salt and freshly ground pepper

1 avocado, peeled and pitted

1 tablespoon fresh lime juice

1 teaspoon tamari

2 tablespoons thinly sliced scallions, white and green parts

2 toasted nori sheets

¼ cup julienned carrots

¼ cup julienned zucchini

¼ cup thinly shaved cabbage

2 tablespoons julienned radishes

1. Preheat the oven to 375°F.

2. Rub the oil over the fish, season with salt and pepper to taste, and arrange on a baking sheet. Bake until slightly opaque and firm to the touch, about 12 minutes depending on thickness. Let cool and break up into pieces (keeping the skin is optional).

3. In a small bowl, smash the avocado slightly with the lime juice, tamari, and scallions (you should have about ¾ cup).

4. Lay the nori sheets on a flat surface and spread a tablespoon or so of the mashed avocado over half of each nori sheet, leaving a ½-inch border on one edge. Press some salmon into the avocado and arrange the carrots, zucchini, cabbage, and radishes on top.

5. Starting with the side with the ½-inch border, roll each nori sheet tightly to enclose the filling, using a dab of water along the last edge so it will stick when closed. Cut each roll into 3 or 4 pieces with a sharp knife.

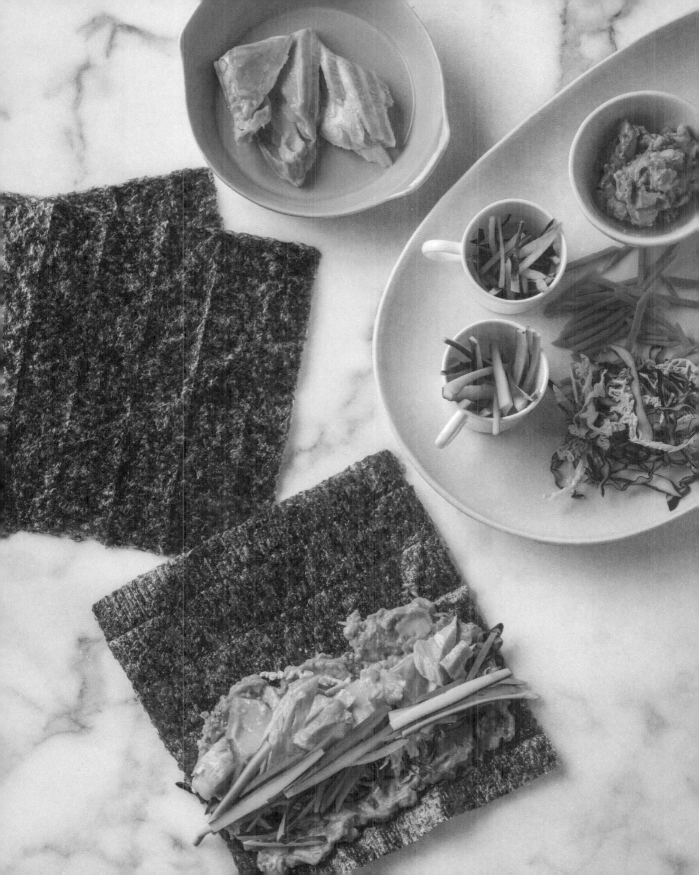

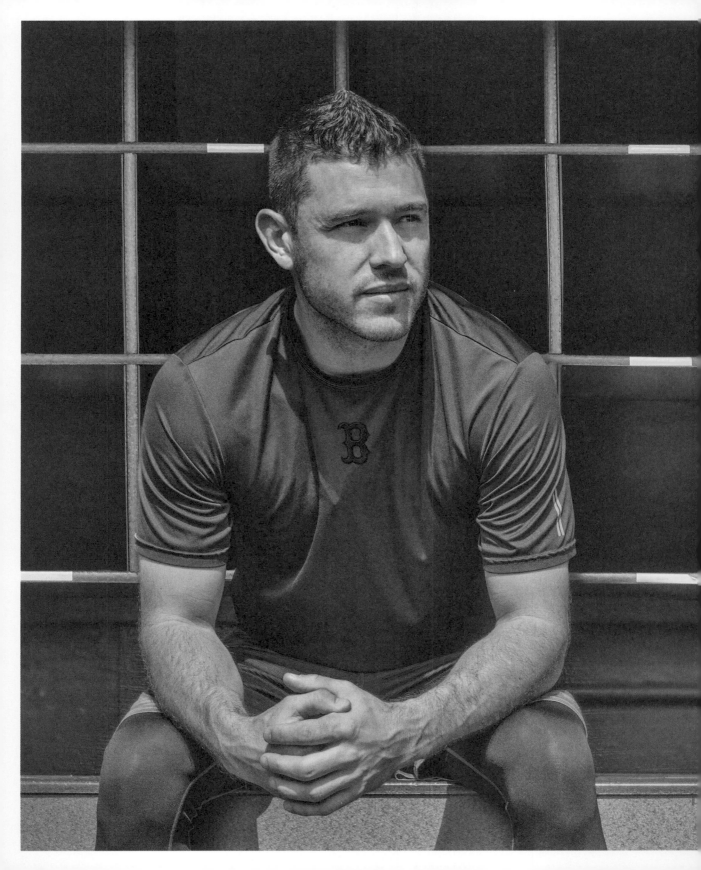

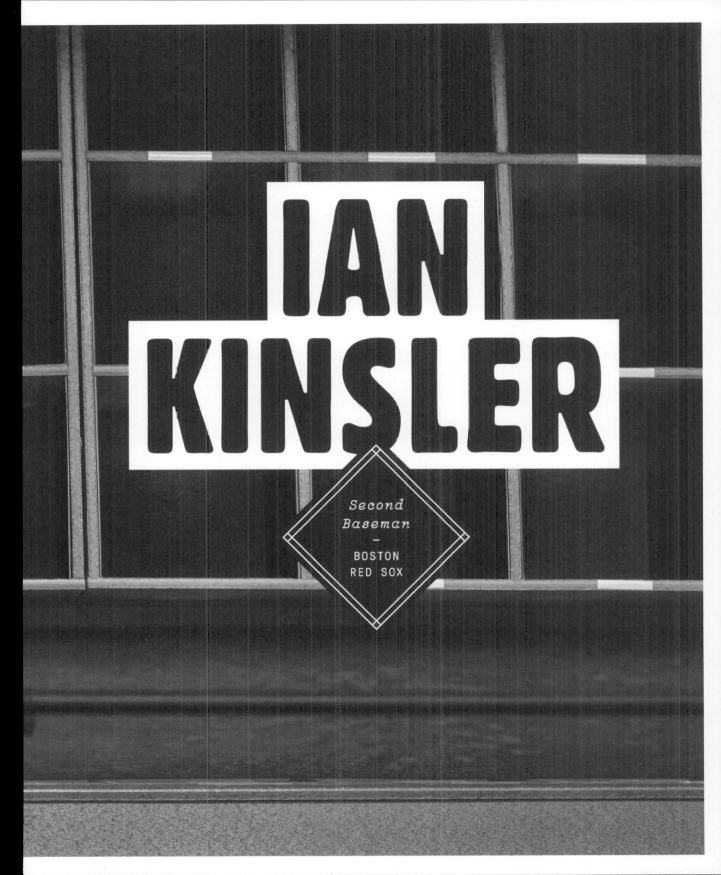

IAN KINSLER

Second
Baseman
—
BOSTON
RED SOX

I've noticed a big change in how I feel during the season—how I eat and take care of myself is constantly evolving as I learn new things. When I played in Texas I didn't know as much as I do now about nutrition and health—how to stay on top of it, and how to keep my energy up. It all kind of started coming together when I got traded to Detroit a few years ago.

I make one cup of Bulletproof coffee in the morning every single day with butter and coconut oil. People look at me like I'm crazy when I drop butter into my coffee, but it works. As I've gotten older, I've found where I need to be physically, and I'm not worried as much about being super strong or heavy, all the things when I was younger that I thought would help me in this game. I'm older now, so I want to be quick. I want to be fast, and I want to stay that way.

Breakfast for me is like grazing—it takes me about thirty minutes to finish breakfast. It's not like I sit down and have everything right in front of me and eat it all at once. I'll have coffee right when I wake up, and I'll eat a bowl of raw oats with some kind of granola mixed in with flax and chia

FULL NAME: Ian Michael Kinsler

HEIGHT/WEIGHT: 6'0", 200 lbs

BORN: June 22, 1982, in Tucson, AZ

POSITION: Second baseman

DRAFT: Drafted by the Arizona Diamondbacks in the 29th round of the 2000 MLB Draft; the Arizona Diamondbacks in the 26th round of the 2001 MLB Draft; and the Texas Rangers in the 17th round of the 2003 MLB Draft

HIGH SCHOOL: Canyon del Oro High School (Oro Valley, AZ)

COLLEGE: Central Arizona College (Coolidge, AZ); Arizona State University (Tempe, AZ); University of Missouri Columbia (Columbia, MO)

AWARDS AND RECOGNITION: 2018 World Series Champion; 4x AL All-Star; 2x AL Gold Glove Award; 2015 Fielding Bible Award; 2x 30-30 Club; hit for the cycle on April 15, 2009

seeds and all that stuff. Then after I'm done with that I kind of mosey around. I'll eat a couple hard-boiled eggs, some vegetables, and then some fruit—just kind of picking.

We always have fresh raspberries and blackberries in our refrigerator. We drive We drive forty-five minutes north of where we live to a farm where you can pick your own fruits and vegetables. We take our kids up there. They love it.

My favorite vegetables are bell peppers, which I love because they're sweet and easy, and I also like broccoli. I always have the refrigerator stocked with vegetables, fruit, and usually a rotisserie chicken because it's an easy food to keep on hand.

My energy snack is local honey. I just take a tablespoon to wake me up and give me energy.

My favorite fresh juice is a hot shot, which has ginger, lemon, and cayenne. I used to never touch ginger, but now I eat it all the time and put it in my drinks and my hot shots. I make a juice with turmeric, grapefruit, and honey. That helps settle my stomach and prevent

> *"I've noticed a big change in how I feel during the season—how I eat and take care of myself is constantly evolving as I learn new things."*

inflammation. And then I'll just pick a random juice every day, like beets, which are good for energy. There's nothing I don't like in the realm of fresh juicing.

As athletes, we're conditioned to think bigger, faster, and stronger, but that's not always ideal. You have to think about how you feel and how your body feels. We're playing 162 games plus Spring Training. If you can keep yourself on the field and stay healthy, you're going to be successful. I've learned that for me it's about how much energy I have and the way I feel. It's not how much I can squat, or how much I can bench. I was the same player, but I didn't feel well. I didn't move well. When I was younger my body could handle it. But then you get to a point where you start to feel lethargic. My off-season workouts have changed drastically. Now I'm driven to

functionality and I'm just trying to keep my body in line. If you put all this weight on your shoulders, and you're doing all these squats, eventually some part of your body is going to get out of line and you're going to be overcompensating for that. I just try to make sure that my body is working properly and that I'm healthy, and the game is going to take care of itself.

I try to keep life as simple as possible. I know what my kids are doing today. I know what my wife is doing today. I know what I'm doing. That's all that matters. My kids help keep things in perspective so much, just wiping all my worries away. You try to perform your best and do everything you can to win, but when it's over, it's over. I have my kids and my family and I'll have them when I can't play this game anymore. That's what keeps me grounded.

ROASTED VEGETABLES

with Sunny-Side Up Eggs

SERVES: *1* // **PREP:** *20 minutes* // **COOK:** *15 minutes*

When it comes to breakfast, Ian Kinsler likes to eat a little of everything, including eggs and vegetables. The combination of the roasted vegetables with the oozing yolk is crazy delicious. The sunny-side up eggs are essential in this dish. They become the ideal sauce for the veggies.

1 cup diced zucchini

1 cup broccoli florets

1 cup diced bell pepper

2½ teaspoons coconut oil, melted

½ teaspoon ground cumin

½ teaspoon ground turmeric

⅛ teaspoon freshly ground black pepper, plus more to taste

Salt

1 tablespoon chopped fresh flat-leaf parsley

2 large eggs

1. Preheat the oven to 425°F.

2. In a large bowl, combine the zucchini, broccoli, bell pepper, 1½ teaspoons of the oil, cumin, turmeric, black pepper, and salt to taste. Arrange the vegetables in a single layer on a baking sheet and roast for 10 to 12 minutes, until golden brown. Add the parsley and toss.

3. In a medium nonstick skillet, heat the remaining 1 teaspoon oil over medium heat. Break the eggs gently into the skillet and cook for 4 to 5 minutes, until the whites are set. Season with salt and pepper to taste. Spoon the roasted veggies into a bowl and top with the eggs.

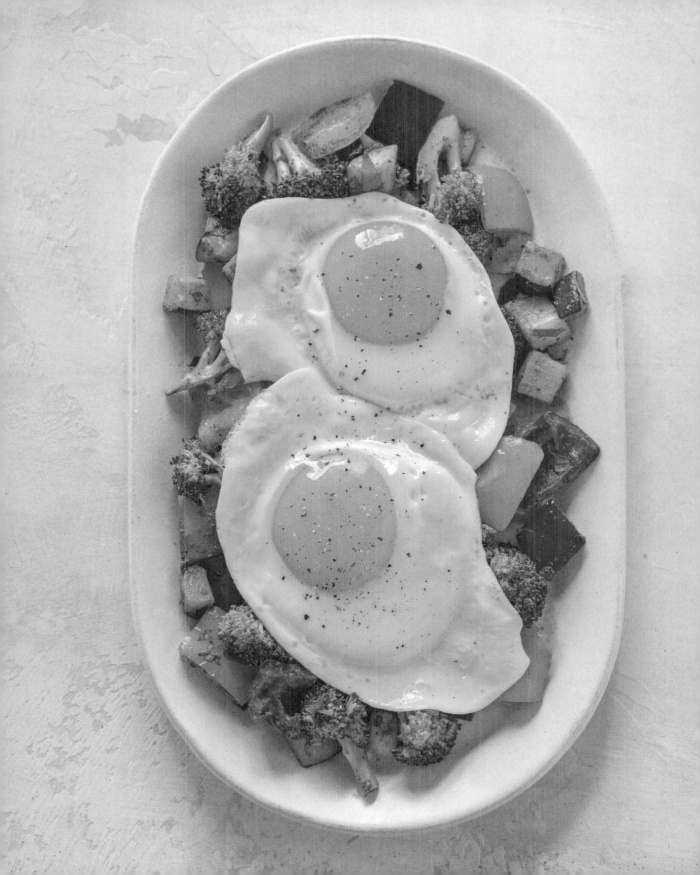

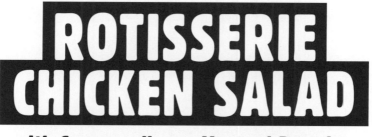

ROTISSERIE CHICKEN SALAD

with Sesame–Honey Mustard Dressing

SERVES: *2* // **PREP:** *15 minutes*

When you're short on time, a rotisserie chicken from your local grocer does the trick for this no-cook chicken salad. The pickled ginger adds a touch of fresh flavor and helps the digestive system too.

8 ounces shredded rotisserie chicken, skin and bones removed

3 cups thinly sliced trimmed bok choy

1 cup julienned daikon radish

2 tablespoons thinly sliced Pickled Ginger (recipe follows)

Sesame–Honey Mustard Dressing (recipe follows)

2 tablespoons chopped fresh mint or cilantro

Salt

2 tablespoons toasted sesame seeds

1. In a large bowl, combine the chicken, bok choy, daikon, and pickled ginger. Fold in the dressing and mint and season with salt to taste.

2. Divide between 2 bowls and top with the sesame seeds.

PICKLED GINGER

SERVES: *2 (makes ¼ cup)* //
PREP: *5 minutes* // **COOK:** *15 minutes*

1 large piece of ginger root, peeled

¼ cup unseasoned rice wine vinegar

¼ teaspoon salt

¼ teaspoon coconut sugar

1. A spoon is the best tool to peel the ginger root. Use a mandoline to slice the ginger as thin as you can; you want ¼ cup.

2. In a small saucepan over medium-low heat, bring the ginger, 1½ cups water, vinegar, salt, and sugar to a simmer. Cook at a slow simmer for 15 minutes.

3. Let cool; then transfer to a jar and store in the refrigerator for up to 3 months.

Note: For a milder, less spicy pickled ginger, blanch the sliced ginger in water first. In a saucepan over medium-high heat, bring 3 inches of water to a boil. Add the sliced ginger and simmer for 1 minute. Strain the water, rinse, and then proceed with step 2 above.

SESAME–HONEY MUSTARD DRESSING

SERVES: *2 (makes ¼ cup)* //
PREP: *5 minutes*

2 tablespoons raw honey

1 tablespoon yellow mustard

1 tablespoon toasted sesame oil

In a small mixing bowl, whisk together the honey, mustard, and toasted sesame oil.

COCONUT MOCHA LATTE

SERVES: *2* // **PREP:** *5 minutes*

A nod to coffee lovers, this latte (pictured on page 67) is super scrumptious and light. The coconut ingredients are a delightful and enticing touch.

1 cup coconut water

¾ cup full-fat canned coconut milk (shake well before measuring)

¼ cup black coffee

1 tablespoon unsweetened cacao powder

1½ teaspoons coconut oil, melted

1 tablespoon maple syrup (optional)

In a high-powered blender, combine the coconut water, milk, coffee, cacao, oil, and syrup (if using) and process until frothy, 45 seconds. Divide between 2 mugs.

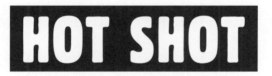

HOT SHOT

SERVES: *2* // **PREP:** *10 minutes*

There is no turning back once you drink this hot juice shot. The combination of the ginger and cayenne makes this drink intensely powerful, but the digestive benefits are endless. Give it a little love and try it.

1 cup chopped ginger root

1 lemon, peel discarded and fruit chopped

2 pinches of cayenne

Pass the ginger and chopped lemon through a juicer. You should have about ⅔ cup of liquid. Divide between 2 glasses and add a pinch of cayenne to each.

GRAPEFRUIT TURMERIC MANUKA SHOT

SERVES: *2* // **PREP:** *10 minutes*

Manuka honey adds a natural sweetness to the tart grapefruit and pungent turmeric in this shot (pictured on page 55). Full of amazing antibacterial and antibiotic medicinal properties, manuka honey is worth every penny.

1¼ cups peeled and chopped ruby red grapefruit

1-inch piece of turmeric root, chopped

½ teaspoon manuka honey

Pinch of freshly ground pepper

Pass the grapefruit and turmeric through a juicer. You should have about ⅔ cup of liquid. Stir in the manuka honey and pepper. Divide between 2 glasses.

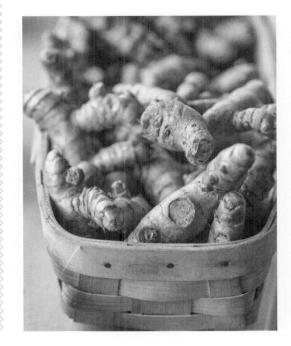

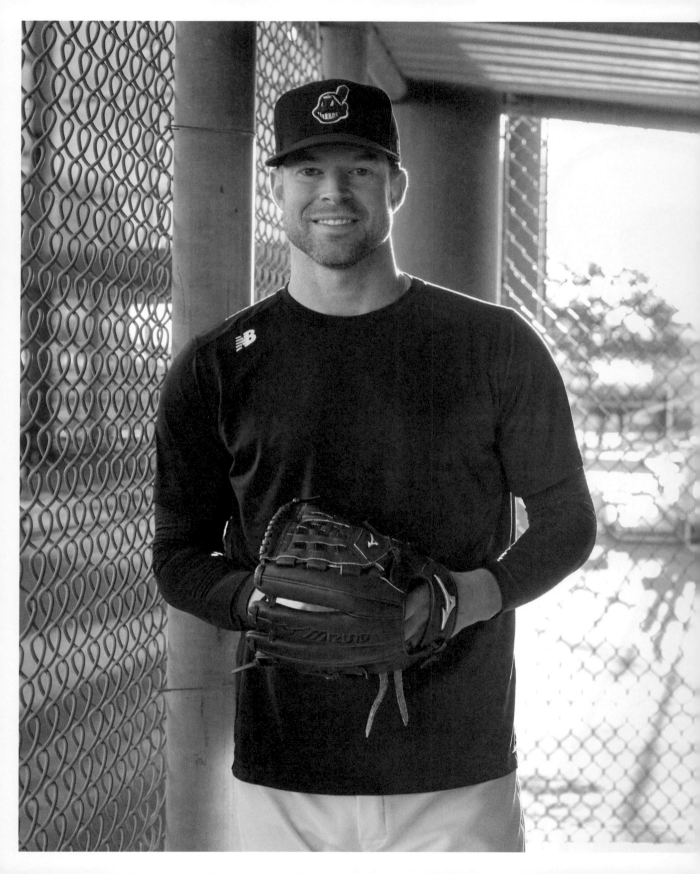

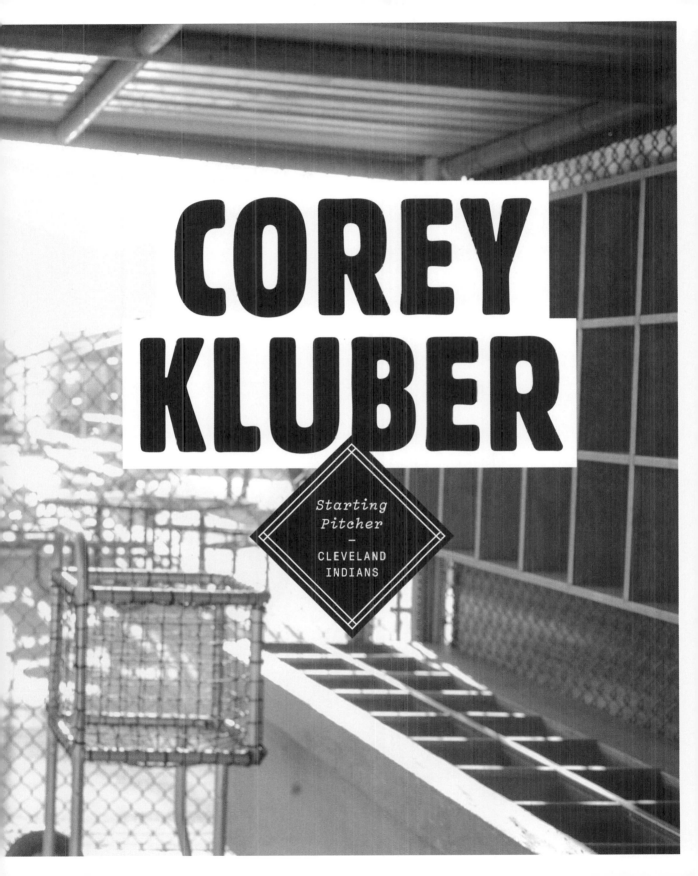

COREY KLUBER

Starting
Pitcher
—
CLEVELAND
INDIANS

Once I started eating better, I started to feel better—it not only improved my energy levels, but my joints felt better. I moved better. This started about five years ago. That was the first time it started to click for me. I noticed a difference in how I felt when I woke up in the morning. I wasn't eating fast food every day, but I wasn't eating particularly well. I didn't make a connection between how I felt and what I ate. I wouldn't say I'm extreme by any means, but I try to pay attention to what I do, and it becomes a habit over time.

I make sure I'm eating food that gives my body the fuel it needs to perform well. I notice how food affects my workouts during the off-season when I'm sitting around watching football and I order a pizza or eat chips and salsa. Getting up that next day and going to work out, I feel the difference from when I've eaten food that's healthy. I've educated myself enough to know what foods are basically good for me and what's not. And I try to lean toward the good.

Breakfast is my biggest meal of the day during Spring Training—I will have an omelet with vegetables in it and an avocado, and then oatmeal with nuts and flaxseeds. During the season if we have a day game and I'm pitching, then breakfast is not my biggest meal.

For lunch I don't zone in on eating the same thing every day. I'm pretty flexible. Some days I might eat a turkey burger or boneless chicken wings with Mexican or Asian flavors just to mix it up. I don't eat a lot of bread. On the days I pitch I eat a pasta with protein and mixed vegetables. Usually it is chicken or shrimp and a vegetable stir-fry.

During the off-season I eat differently, and my wife and I do a lot of the cooking. If I'm home on an off-season day, I usually make eggs, but if I'm going to the gym and I'm pressed for time, I just make a protein shake.

My energy snack is a small smoothie with frozen berries, fresh-squeezed orange juice, peanut butter, yogurt, oatmeal, and protein powder. I also eat nuts from the clubhouse.

My favorite vegetables are asparagus, Brussels sprouts, and broccoli with olive oil and salt and pepper— all roasted. I could eat a plate full of vegetables every day.

FULL NAME: Corey Scott Kluber

HEIGHT/WEIGHT: 6'4", 215 lbs

BORN: April 10, 1986, in Birmingham, AL

POSITION: Pitcher

DRAFT: Drafted by the San Diego Padres in the 4th round of the 2007 MLB Draft

HIGH SCHOOL: Coppell High School (Coppell, TX)

COLLEGE: Stetson University (DeLand, FL)

AWARDS AND RECOGNITION: 3x AL All-Star; 2x AL Cy Young Award; 2x AL wins leader; 2017 AL ERA leader

"I've educated myself enough to know what foods are basically good for me and what's not. And I try to lean toward the good."

During the off-season dinner is some sort of protein like salmon with vegetables and a carb, usually pasta, quinoa, or couscous. My wife and I cook together probably half of the week.

I recently discovered that I like avocados. I eat them plain, in guacamole, on a turkey burger, or in an omelet.

The best wellness advice I've received is that health is about finding balance. It's not the worst thing in the world to have a slice of pizza, as long as it's in moderation. I allow myself to eat things that are unhealthy. But more often than not, I try to choose healthy foods.

Wellness is made up of different pieces of a puzzle: Food is a piece, working out is a piece, and family is a piece. Working out is my meditation and training for my brain, so to speak. It stimulates my mind.

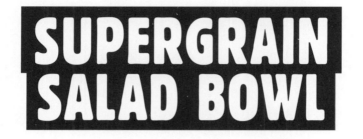

SUPERGRAIN SALAD BOWL

SERVES: *2* // **PREP:** *20 minutes* // **COOK:** *20 minutes*

Grain salads are nutritious and filling without weighing you down. This undeniably good, nutrient-dense recipe is so satisfying as a lunch or dinner. Be sure to save any leftovers for a really quick next-day meal.

2 cups broccoli florets

½ cup peas (frozen peas are great for this)

2 cups diced sweet potato, unpeeled

2 tablespoons finely chopped shallots

1½ teaspoons coconut oil, melted

Salt and freshly ground pepper

1 cup cooked quinoa, warm (see page 13)

1 cup cooked millet, warm (see page 13)

2 tablespoons fresh lemon juice

2 teaspoons chopped fresh thyme

1. Preheat the oven to 400°F.

2. In a saucepan fitted with a steamer basket, bring 1 inch of water to a boil. Put the broccoli in the basket, cover, and steam for 1½ minutes. Drain well and transfer to a large bowl. Set aside.

3. In a saucepan fitted with a steamer basket, bring 1 inch of water to a boil. Put the peas in the basket, cover, and steam for 1 minute. Drain well and transfer to a large bowl. Set aside. For frozen peas, spread in an even layer on a dish, and let thaw for 15 to 20 minutes before steaming.

4. In a medium bowl, combine the sweet potato, shallots, and oil. Season with salt and pepper to taste and spread in an even layer on a baking sheet. Bake for 16 to 18 minutes, until the potatoes are tender.

5. Add the sweet potato to the bowl with the broccoli along with the quinoa, millet, peas, lemon juice, and thyme. Season with salt and pepper to taste. Divide between 2 bowls.

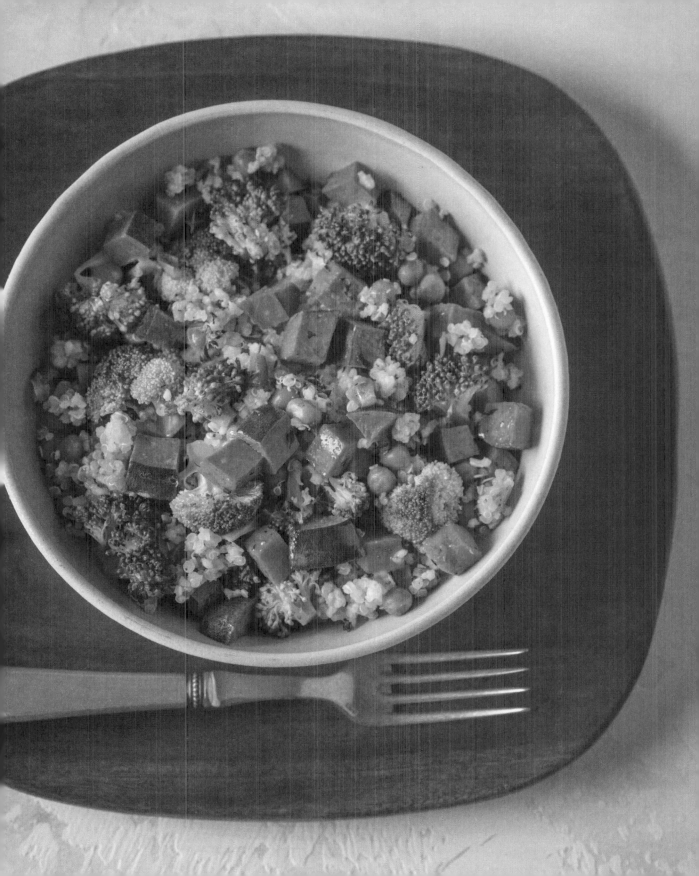

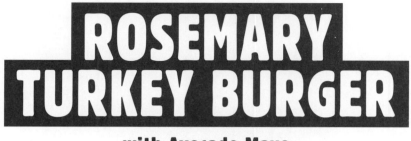

ROSEMARY TURKEY BURGER

with Avocado Mayo

SERVES: 2 // **PREP:** 20 minutes // **COOK:** 25 minutes

These easy turkey burgers are a must. The walnuts and rosemary bring the burger flavors to a new level. Serve with the simple-to-make avocado mayo for the ultimate burger condiment.

½ cup walnuts

1 tablespoon plus 1 teaspoon coconut oil, melted

¼ cup finely chopped yellow onion

8 ounces ground turkey (white and dark meat)

2 teaspoons chopped fresh rosemary

⅛ teaspoon crushed red pepper flakes

½ teaspoon salt

4 cups salad greens

2 cups sliced cucumber

1 lemon, halved

¼ cup Avocado Mayo (recipe follows on page 180)

1. Preheat the oven to 375°F.

2. Arrange the walnuts in a single layer on a baking sheet and toast for 8 to 10 minutes. Remove from the oven and let cool. In a food processor, chop the nuts until coarsely ground, about 10 seconds.

3. Heat the 1 teaspoon oil in a skillet over medium heat. Add the onion and cook, stirring, until golden brown, about 3 minutes. Let cool.

4. In a medium bowl, combine the turkey, ground walnuts, rosemary, red pepper flakes, salt, and cooled onion. Shape into 2 burgers. Heat the remaining 1 tablespoon oil in a medium skillet over medium heat until hot but not smoking. Cook the burgers until golden brown and cooked through, 4 to 5 minutes per side.

5. Divide the greens and cucumber between 2 bowls and squeeze a lemon half over the top of each portion. Add a turkey burger to each bowl and serve with avocado mayo.

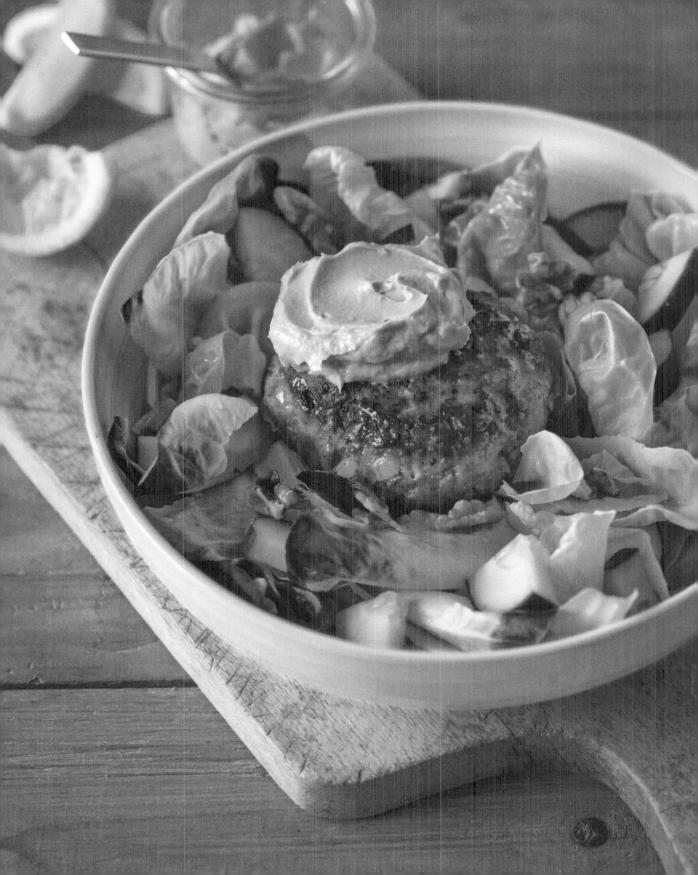

AVOCADO MAYO

MAKES: *1½ cups* // **PREP:** *5 minutes*

**2 ripe avocados, halved, pitted, and flesh
scooped out with a spoon**

1½ teaspoons fresh lemon juice

¼ teaspoon grated garlic

Salt and freshly ground pepper

Combine the avocados, lemon, and garlic in a
high-speed blender and process until smooth.
Season with salt and pepper to taste. Store in
an airtight container in the refrigerator for up
to 2 days.

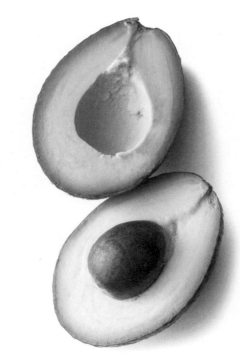

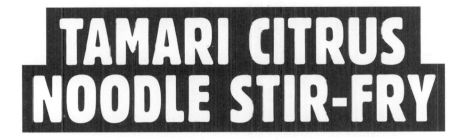

TAMARI CITRUS NOODLE STIR-FRY

SERVES: *4* // **PREP:** *20 minutes* // **COOK:** *5 minutes*

Tamari and rice noodles help make this veggie stir-fry light and luscious, and the blend of citrus, garlic, herbs, and spices is spot-on.

2 tablespoons tamari

1 tablespoon fresh lime juice

1 tablespoon fresh lemon juice

3 cups thinly sliced trimmed bok choy

½ cup julienned daikon radish

½ cup julienned carrots

½ cup drained canned sliced water chestnuts

¼ cup thinly sliced scallions, white and green parts

1½ teaspoons grated garlic

1½ teaspoons grated ginger

4 ounces brown rice noodles

1 tablespoon toasted sesame oil

1½ teaspoons coconut oil

2 tablespoons chopped fresh mint (optional)

2 tablespoons chopped fresh cilantro (optional)

1 tablespoon toasted sesame seeds

4 lime wedges, for serving

1. In a small bowl, whisk the tamari, lime and lemon juices, and 1 tablespoon water. Set aside.

2. In a large bowl, combine the bok choy, daikon, carrots, water chestnuts, scallions, garlic, and ginger. Toss until all the vegetables are evenly coated in garlic and ginger.

3. Cook the rice noodles according to the package directions. Rinse, drain well, and toss in the toasted sesame seed oil.

4. Heat the coconut oil in a large skillet over high heat. Cook the vegetables, stirring continuously, for just 10 seconds. Remove from the heat and toss in the rice noodles, reserved tamari citrus sauce, and herbs (if using). Divide between 2 bowls. Top with sesame seeds and serve with lime wedges.

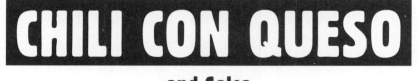

CHILI CON QUESO
and Salsa

SERVES: *6* // **PREP:** *15 minutes*

This rich and creamy nondairy "cheese" dip is so over-the-moon good you'll be making it again and again. The bold flavors pair beautifully with salsa. Together they can be served with a side of raw veggies or organic corn tortilla chips for a healthful, crowd-pleasing snack.

1 cup raw cashews (If not using a high-powered blender, soak the cashews for 8 hours or up to 12 hours in room-temperature water. Drain and rinse well.)

2 red bell peppers, roasted, skin and seeds removed (see Tomato Sauce on page 96)

¼ cup fresh lemon juice

3 tablespoons nutritional yeast

1 teaspoon salt

½ teaspoon crushed red pepper flakes, or to taste

In a high-powered blender, combine all ingredients with 2 tablespoons water and process until smooth.

SALSA

1½ cups diced tomato

½ cup diced bell pepper

¼ cup finely chopped red onion

½ teaspoon grated garlic

1 tablespoon extra-virgin olive oil

1 tablespoon fresh lime juice

1 tablespoon chopped fresh cilantro

1 teaspoon minced seeded jalapeño

Salt and freshly ground pepper

In a medium bowl, combine all ingredients through the jalapeño. Season with salt and pepper to taste.

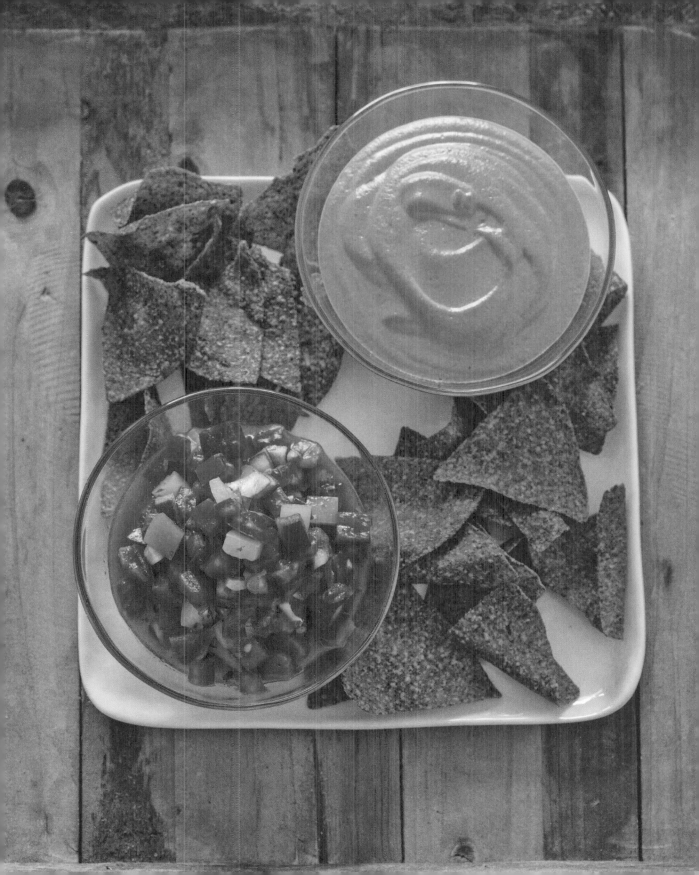

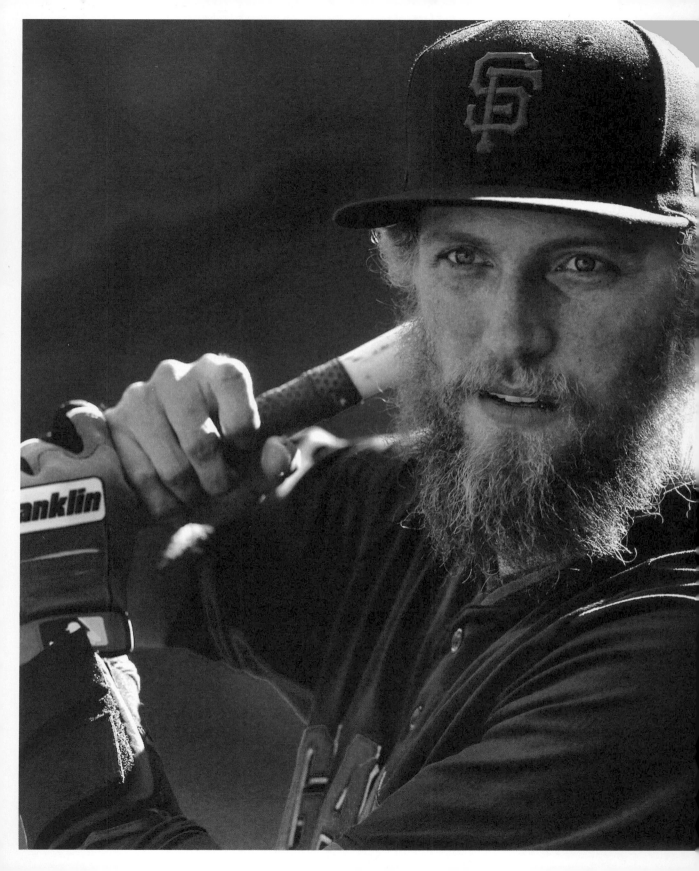

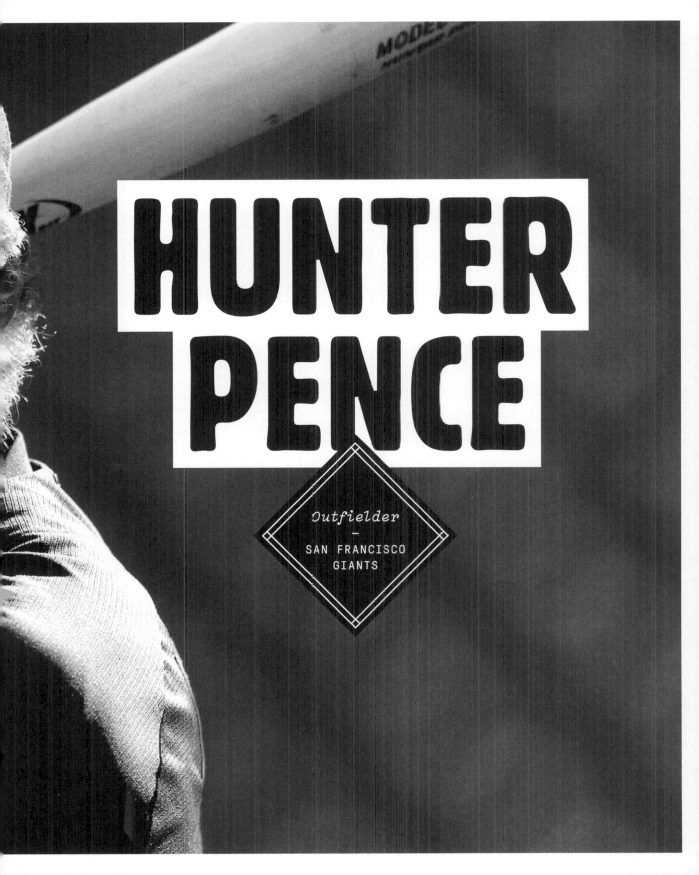

HUNTER PENCE

Outfielder
—
SAN FRANCISCO GIANTS

My motivation to eat smart is a desire to give my best on the field. I'm grateful to play the game so I try to find every opportunity to give my best out there. If eating better is going to help me play better or feel better, that's very important to me.

I saw the connection between eating better and playing better when I was coming up from college. I always dreamed of being a Major Leaguer. I knew that how you fuel your body improves how you feel on the field. I was extremely skinny in high school, so I started studying what to eat to gain weight. As I got older I wanted to fuel my body the right way.

During the off-season I follow a paleo diet. Back when I had just joined the Giants, my brother and I read a book about it and I started trying it. When I started eating kale, I was teased a lot. Kale wasn't popular yet, but then the other players caught on, and it inspired our team president and his wife to build an edible garden in the outfield. It's called Hunter's Garden. Honestly, when I follow a paleo diet, I feel the best I ever have, but it's virtually impossible to do during the baseball season because we travel so much.

FULL NAME: Hunter Andrew Pence

HEIGHT/WEIGHT: 6'4", 215 lbs

BORN: April 13, 1983, in Fort Worth, TX

POSITION: Right fielder

DRAFT: Drafted by the Milwaukee Brewers in the 40th round of the 2002 MLB Draft and the Houston Astros in the 2nd round of the 2004 MLB Draft

HIGH SCHOOL: Arlington High School (Arlington, TX)

COLLEGE: Texarkana College (Texarkana, TX); University of Texas at Arlington (Arlington, TX)

AWARDS AND RECOGNITION: 2x World Series Champion; 3x NL All-Star; 2013 Willie Mac Award; 2008 Darryl Kile Award

My breakfast includes açai bowls. I really love them. I'll eat one of those with a Bulletproof coffee. My wife learned how to make paleo pancakes out of bananas. She smashes them up with eggs and makes pancakes. It's really cool. I even add kale to my breakfast from time to time.

Every day I eat vegetables. If I don't have vegetables I won't feel well. That's why I love kale so much. I also like bell peppers and avocado. I could eat those every day and feel good.

My energy snack is a banana or a protein bar. I eat them all the time during games. I get hungry. On the road I drink a lot of protein shakes, and I'll throw in kale, cauliflower, and broccoli and make a pure veggie smoothie. Occasionally I'll use almond milk in my smoothies too.

The fruit I eat the most is bananas. I wouldn't say I can't live without them, but they're the most convenient and easy snack. I try not to eat tons of fruits because of the sugar content.

To help speed muscle recovery after a tough workout, I make sure to rest. Sleeping and making sure I'm eating my vegetables and hydrating. That's all I focus on.

> *"My motivation to eat smart is a desire to give my best on the field. I'm grateful to play the game so I try to find every opportunity to give my best out there. If eating better is going to help me play better or feel better, that's very important to me."*

My biggest meal of the day is probably dinner—I'll have salmon with a nice spinach and kale salad and some sweet potatoes. I eat a big breakfast too, though. It just depends on how hungry I am. Usually, when I'm playing, I'll eat a huge meal after the game; I don't eat that much right before the game. I want to have a light stomach.

Besides eating smart, my support for living smart comes from nature. Time in nature can nurture anyone. Or quiet time spent anywhere, just to fill your spirit.

CHERRY AÇAI BOWL

SERVES: *1* // PREP: *5 minutes*

Every spoonful of this outrageously gorgeous bowl is full of flavor thanks to the healthy goodness of the antioxidant-rich açai. Add a topping of your choice, such as berries, seeds, and nuts, for some extra nutritional flavor and crunch.

1 (3.5-ounce) package frozen açai
2 to 4 tablespoons coconut water
1 medium very ripe banana, sliced
½ cup frozen pitted dark cherries
½ cup frozen wild blueberries

TOPPING SUGGESTIONS
¼ cup Green Monster Crunch (page 201)
½ cup berries, nuts, and seeds

1. Break up the frozen sealed açai pack on a hard surface to help it blend smoothly. In a high-powered blender, combine the açai, 2 tablespoons coconut water, banana, cherries, and blueberries. Process until smooth, adding additional coconut water if necessary to facilitate blending.

2. Spoon into a bowl and add your favorite toppings.

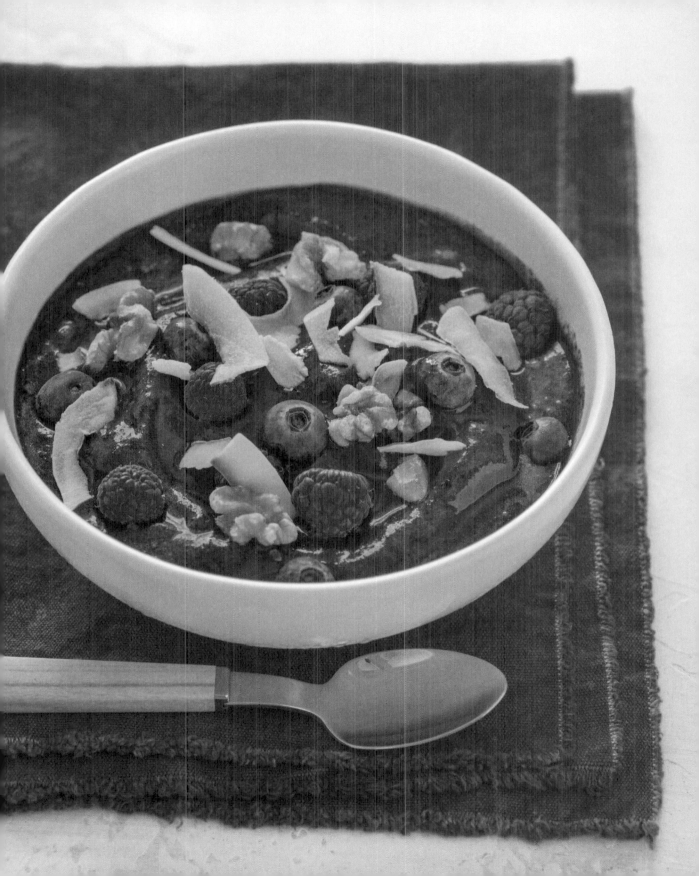

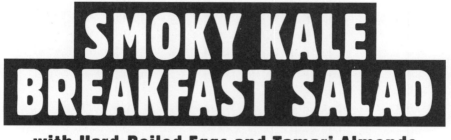

SMOKY KALE BREAKFAST SALAD

with Hard-Boiled Eggs and Tamari Almonds

SERVES: *2* // **PREP:** *15 minutes* // **COOK:** *15 minutes*

Who says breakfast has to be sweet all the time? This quick and easy twist on simply prepared eggs is an unexpected breakfast pleasure. The tamari almonds add a great crunchy texture.

2 large eggs

2 cups thinly sliced curly kale, tough ribs removed first

½ cup thinly sliced bell pepper

½ cup chopped broccoli florets

2 tablespoons fresh lemon juice

1 tablespoon torn basil

2 tablespoons chopped tamari almonds

⅛ teaspoon smoked salt

Freshly ground pepper

2 tablespoons extra-virgin olive oil

1. Put the eggs in a saucepan and cover with water by at least 2 inches. Bring to a boil and cook for 1 minute. Remove from heat, cover tightly, and let sit for 12 minutes. Drain the eggs and cool them down in a bowl of ice water. As you start to peel, continue to dip the eggs into the bowl of ice water as needed. (This makes the shells slip off more easily.) Slice evenly, and set aside.

2. In a large bowl, combine the kale, bell pepper, broccoli, lemon juice, and basil.

3. Divide the kale salad into 2 bowls, each topped with a sliced egg. Sprinkle each bowl with the tamari almonds, smoked salt, and black pepper to taste. Drizzle olive oil over the top.

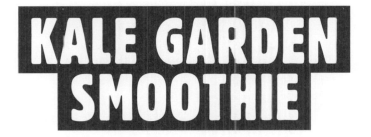

KALE GARDEN SMOOTHIE

SERVES: *1* // **PREP:** *10 minutes*

Hunter Pence loves kale so much he inspired the creation of the first-ever ballpark kale garden. The leafy green is a welcome dimension to this super-tasty and slightly sweet smoothie.

1½ cups chilled aloe water

1 cup baby kale

1 banana, broken into pieces

1-inch piece of ginger root, chopped

1-inch piece of turmeric root, chopped

½ lemon, peel discarded and fruit chopped

1 tablespoon coconut oil, melted (optional)

A few ice cubes (optional)

In a high-powered blender, combine all ingredients, using coconut oil and ice if desired, and process until smooth.

BANANA PANCAKES

SERVES: *4 (makes about twelve 3- to 4-inch pancakes)*
PREP: *10 minutes* // **COOK:** *15 minutes*

Ripe and ready bananas provide a natural sweetness to these deliciously good gluten-free, dairy-free pancakes. Before cooking, be sure to let the batter rest for 10 minutes to achieve pancake perfection. The texture will be slightly different from that of traditional pancakes, but the flavor will be so irresistible you might even skip the syrup—if not, a dark amber pure maple syrup is best.

2 cups sliced very ripe bananas (about 2½ medium)

3 large eggs

3 to 4 tablespoons coconut flour

⅛ teaspoon baking powder

¼ teaspoon ground cinnamon (optional)

¼ teaspoon vanilla extract (optional)

Pinch of salt

4½ teaspoons coconut oil

Fresh berries and pure maple syrup, for topping (optional)

1. In a high-powered blender, combine the bananas, eggs, 3 tablespoons coconut flour, baking powder, cinnamon, vanilla (if using), and salt and process until smooth. Add the remaining 1 tablespoon flour if the batter is too thin. Let the batter stand for 10 minutes.

2. In a large nonstick skillet set over medium heat, melt 1½ teaspoons of the oil, tilting the pan so it spreads evenly. Ladle 4 pancakes (about ¼ cup each) onto the hot pan and cook for 2 to 3 minutes on each side until golden brown, adjusting the heat as necessary. Repeat with the remaining oil and batter. Serve with your favorite toppings, if desired.

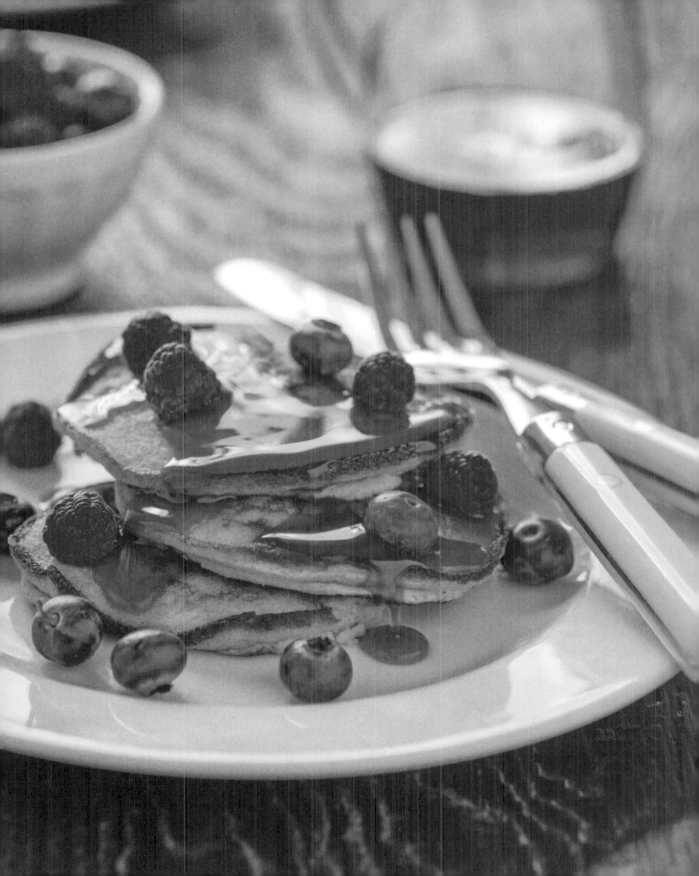

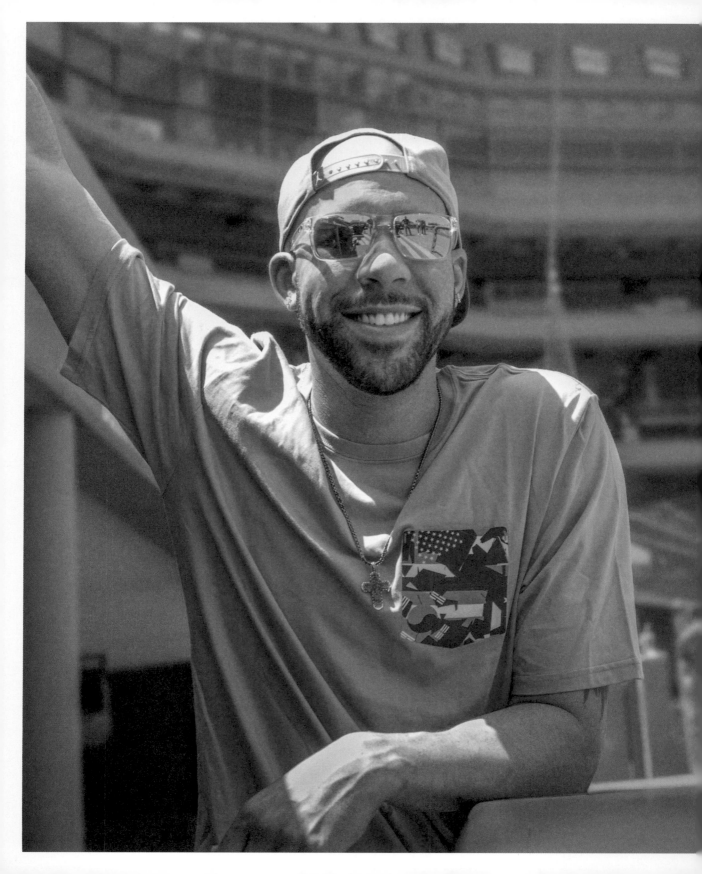

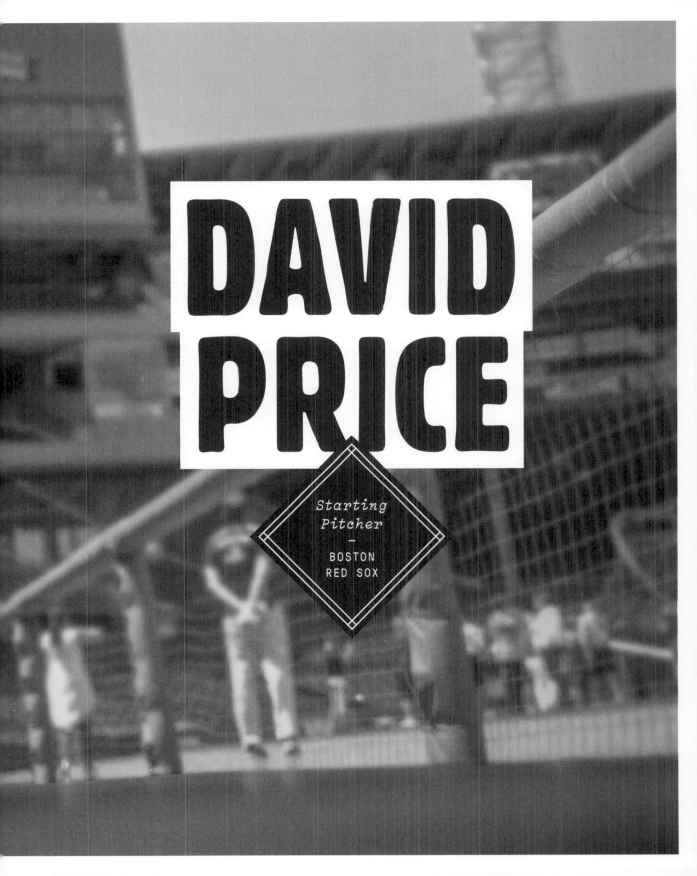

DAVID PRICE

Starting Pitcher

—

BOSTON
RED SOX

My former teammate Gabe Kapler really motivated me to eat smart— he's a stickler about eating for performance and recovery. He got me on almond butter. That was something he was always eating after batting practice to refuel. Just watching the way he went about his work and his nutrition, and seeing the shape that he was in at his age, opened my eyes. It made me start watching what I put in my body and start eating the good stuff, especially two or three nights before I pitch. He always encouraged me to try new things in my diet. I used to be more cut and dry with what I would and wouldn't eat, but trying new things and discovering that I actually enjoy eating healthy food was a big revelation.

I love sweets, but I feel sluggish the next morning if I've had dessert the night before. I see a clear connection between my healthier eating habits and my performance, because I wake up feeling better when I've eaten well.

I love food. I want to enjoy what I eat. To know that I can enjoy food and also eat well was eye-opening. My wife is a healthy eater and she cooks food that's all natural and

FULL NAME: David Taylor Price

HEIGHT/WEIGHT: 6'5", 215 lbs

BORN: August 26, 1985, in Murfreesboro, TN

POSITION: Pitcher

DRAFT: Drafted by the Los Angeles Dodgers in the 19th round of the 2004 MLB Draft and the Tampa Bay Devil Rays in the 1st round (1st) of the 2007 MLB Draft

HIGH SCHOOL: Blackmon High School (Murfreesboro, TN)

COLLEGE: Vanderbilt University (Nashville, TN)

AWARDS AND RECOGNITION: 2018 World Series Champion; 5x AL All-Star; 2012 AL Cy Young Award; 2012 AL wins leader; 2x AL ERA leader; 2014 AL strikeout leader

organic. She turned me on to eating healthy food that is also delicious.

My wife makes homemade all-natural pasta sauce with ground turkey— switching from ground beef to ground turkey was a big change. We use ground turkey now in tacos and pasta; I used to just have store-bought sauce with meat in it.

I try to eat some fruit every day, often in a smoothie because they are so easy to make and take on the go. For an energy snack I have almond butter on apples and bananas. I also drink fresh juices—if it's going to benefit my health, then I'm going to drink it. One of my teammates made me one with beets, kale, all that stuff.

To stay hydrated I drink four bottles of water over the first five innings of pitching. I also have it first thing when I wake up and then have two more bottles in the morning. There's always water on my nightstand, and I load up my backpack when I head to the field. I make sure I'm always hydrated.

I'm always extremely hungry when I finish a game, and usually have

> *"I love sweets, but I feel sluggish the next morning if I've had dessert the night before. I see a clear connection between my healthier eating habits and my performance, because I wake up feeling better when I've eaten well."*

something like sea bass or chicken with brown rice and mixed vegetables. Lunch is usually lighter—I'll have a smoothie for lunch, a protein shake. I'll definitely have something, but it's usually a liquid meal or something with a protein post batting practice.

To me, the best thing about baseball is all the different relationships you build throughout your career. I've made a lot of great friends from all the teams I've played on. I get to meet new guys, whether at an All-Star game or at an off-season event. Baseball is not something I'm going to be able to do forever. At some point, it's going to stop for me, but those friendships are the things I'll take to the grave and what I cherish most.

ROASTED SEA BASS

with Cauliflower Puree

SERVES: *2* // **PREP:** *5 minutes* // **COOK:** *15 minutes*

Cauliflower puree is the MVP of this dish, and the perfect complement to the roasted sea bass. You'll find it hard not to go back for seconds, so you may want to make extra. And remember your greens—the steamed chard completes the meal.

2 (4-ounce) sea bass fillets

½ teaspoon coconut oil, melted

½ teaspoon ground cumin

Salt and freshly ground pepper

Cauliflower Puree and Chard (recipe follows)

1. Preheat the oven to 375°F.

2. Place the fish on a small baking sheet and rub with the oil. Season with the cumin and salt and pepper to taste. Bake until opaque and cooked through, 12 to 15 minutes, depending on thickness.

3. Serve the fish with the cauliflower and chard.

CAULIFLOWER PUREE AND CHARD

SERVES: *2* // **PREP:** *20 minutes* // **COOK:** *30 minutes*

½ cup chopped white onion

1 teaspoon coconut oil, melted

4 cups chopped cauliflower florets

1 tablespoon extra-virgin olive oil

3 cups chopped Swiss chard leaves (any color), ribs removed first

1 lemon wedge

Salt and freshly ground pepper

1. Preheat the oven to 425°F.

2. Toss the onion with the coconut oil and spread in a single layer on a small baking sheet. Roast, stirring once, until just beginning to char, about 10 minutes.

3. Meanwhile, in a saucepan fitted with a steamer basket, bring 3 inches of water to a boil. Put the cauliflower in the basket, cover, and steam for 18 to 20 minutes, until very soft. Combine the cauliflower, onion, and olive oil in a high-speed blender and process until smooth. Season with salt and pepper to taste.

4. Put the chard in a steamer basket, cover, and steam for 15 to 20 seconds, until just wilted. Squeeze the lemon wedge over chard and season with salt.

The Game of Eating Smart

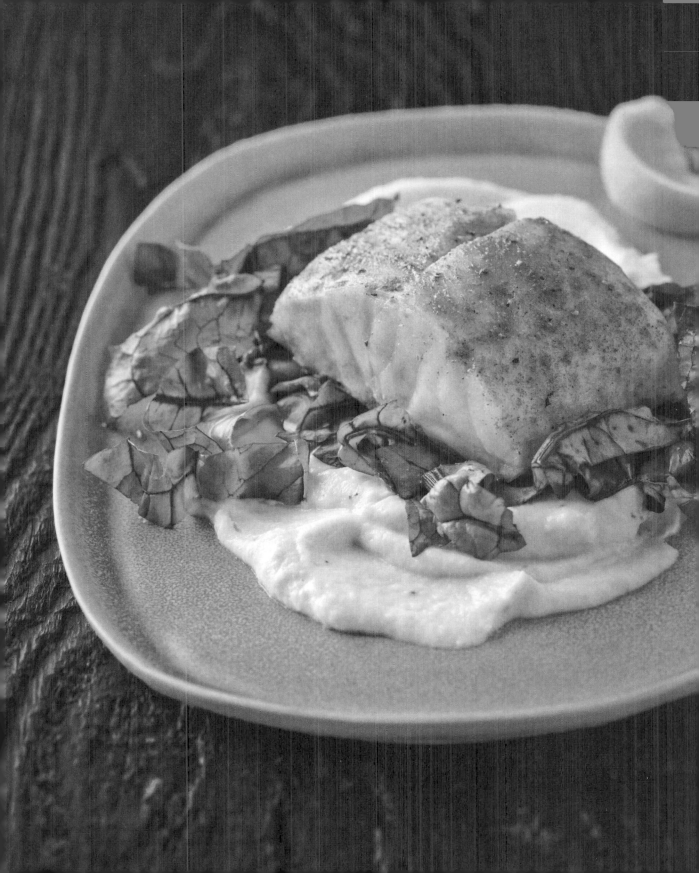

SPICY TOMATO BASIL RICE BOWL

SERVES: *2* // **PREP:** *10 minutes* // **COOK:** *10 minutes*

The next time you crave a wholesome meatless main meal, this nourishing grain bowl will not let you down. Grab a fork and dig in.

2 plum tomatoes, cut into chunks

1 teaspoon avocado oil

½ teaspoon paprika

¼ teaspoon grated garlic

⅛ teaspoon crushed red pepper flakes

Salt and freshly ground pepper

2 cups broccoli florets

3 cups baby arugula

2 cups cooked short-grain brown rice, warm (see page 13)

8 basil leaves, torn

1½ teaspoons fresh lemon juice

1. Preheat the oven to 425°F.

2. In a medium bowl, toss the tomatoes with the oil, paprika, garlic, red pepper flakes, and salt and pepper to taste. Transfer to a casserole dish and roast, stirring once, until golden brown, 10 to 12 minutes.

3. Meanwhile, in a saucepan fitted with a steamer basket, bring 1 inch of water to a boil. Put the broccoli in the basket, cover, and steam for 1 minute. Remove from heat and season with salt.

4. Scrape the roasted tomatoes into a large bowl. Immediately toss with the arugula, rice, broccoli, basil, and lemon juice. Season with salt and pepper to taste. Divide between 2 bowls.

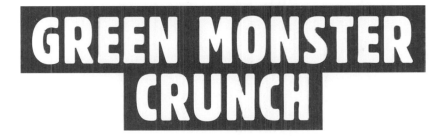

GREEN MONSTER CRUNCH

SERVES: *6* // **PREP:** *5 minutes, plus 2 hours soaking time* // **COOK:** *20 minutes*

This sensational granola is so good it'll knock your (Red) socks off. Grab a handful of crunchy bits when the snack cravings hit you or use it as a topping for coconut yogurt, soup, or a smoothie. Make a bunch and store in an airtight container.

1 cup Brazil nuts

3 cups unsweetened coconut flakes

1 cup walnuts

¼ cup honey

1½ tablespoons coconut oil, melted

2 teaspoons chlorella powder

1. Place the Brazil nuts in a bowl and cover with room-temperature water; soak for 2 hours. Drain well, rinse, and coarsely chop.

2. Preheat the oven to 350°F. Line a baking sheet with a silicone mat.

3. In a food processor, pulse the Brazil nuts, coconut flakes, and walnuts for 10 seconds. Transfer to a large bowl and stir in the honey and oil. Arrange in a single layer on the lined sheet pan and bake for about 20 minutes, stirring every 6 minutes, until golden brown.

4. Return the granola to the large bowl, add the chlorella, and toss until it sticks. Let cool before serving; it will get crunchier as it sits. The granola will keep in an airtight container in the refrigerator for up to 6 weeks.

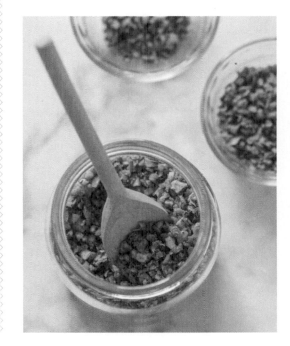

TURKEY TACO BOWL

with Pickled Red Onion

SERVES: *2* // **PREP:** *20 minutes* // **COOK:** *5 minutes*

Taco bowls have all the familiar spicy and savory flavors minus the shell. Any extra pickled onion keeps for up to 4 weeks refrigerated and can be used as a terrific condiment.

1 teaspoon coconut oil

2 tablespoons finely chopped onion

8 ounces ground turkey (mix of white and dark meat)

½ teaspoon ground cumin

½ teaspoon chili powder

⅛ teaspoon cayenne

1½ teaspoons extra-virgin olive oil

Salt and freshly ground pepper

1½ cups cooked short-grain brown rice, warm (see page 13)

2 cups thinly sliced dinosaur kale, tough stems removed first

1 avocado, cut into chunks

¼ cup Pickled Red Onion (recipe follows)

Juice of 1 lime

1. In a medium skillet, heat the coconut oil over medium heat. Cook the onion, stirring, until softened, about 2 minutes. Add the turkey and cook, using a wooden spoon to break it up, until cooked through and no pink remains, about 3 minutes. Stir in the cumin, chili powder, cayenne, olive oil, and salt and pepper to taste.

2. Divide the rice, kale, turkey, avocado, and pickled red onion between 2 bowls. Drizzle with lime juice.

PICKLED RED ONION

MAKES: *about 1¼ cups* // **PREP:** *10 minutes, plus 1 hour marinating time* // **COOK:** *5 minutes*

¾ cup red wine vinegar

¼ cup cider vinegar

2 garlic cloves, smashed

1 teaspoon salt

1 bay leaf

½ teaspoon whole black peppercorns

2 cups thinly shaved red onion

1. In a medium saucepan over medium heat, bring 3 cups water, both vinegars, garlic, salt, bay leaf, and peppercorns to a boil. Reduce the heat to low and simmer for 5 minutes. Put the red onion in a heatproof glass container (like a large mason jar) big enough to hold the liquid; strain the hot liquid over the onions. Let stand for at least 1 hour.

2. Once they've cooled to room temperature, store the onions in the refrigerator in an airtight container for up to 4 weeks. You can strain the liquid if you want to stop the pickling process.

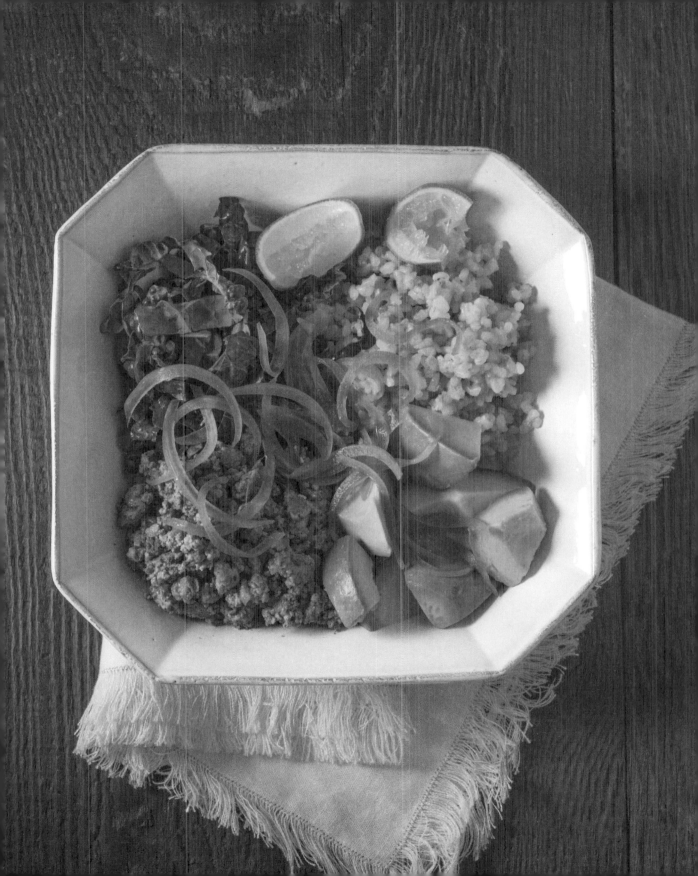

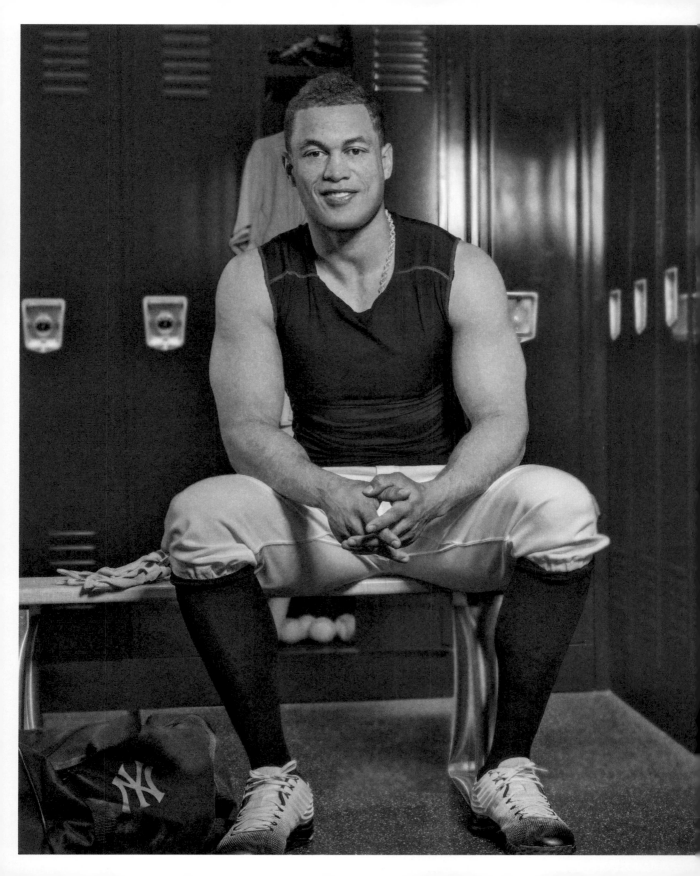

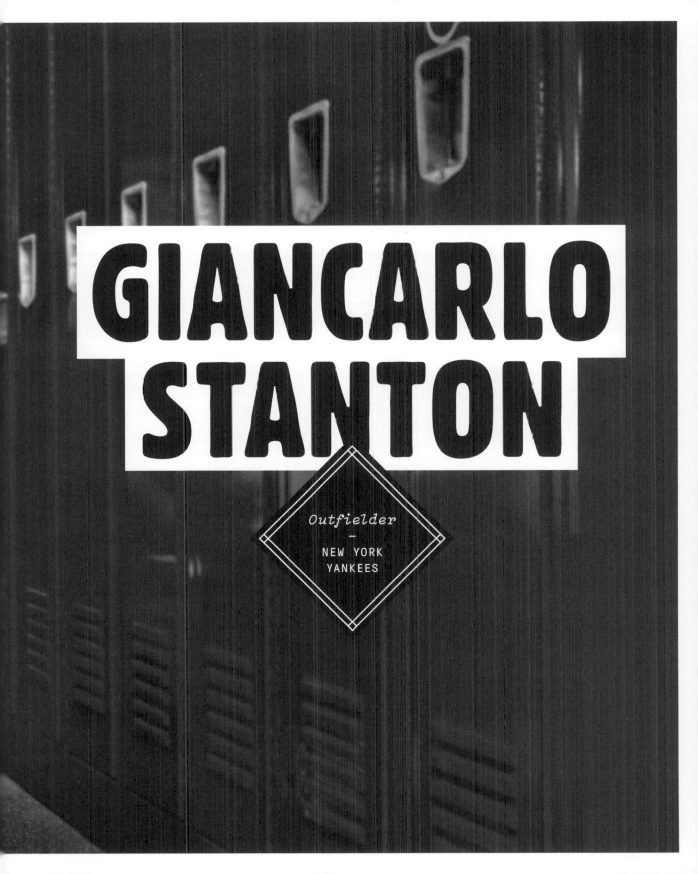

GIANCARLO STANTON

Outfielder
–
NEW YORK
YANKEES

I feel the difference in my body when I wake up or when I have to do physical activity all day after I have eaten poorly. If I don't eat right I feel like I am dragging, especially when I have a couple of bad meals after eating right for an extended period. I feel the difference for sure.

My breakfast is a veggie shake or some protein, so my metabolism and body are working the right way in the morning. I don't have much of a routine other than just keeping my diet clean. I don't like to eat until a few hours after I wake up because I'm not hungry. So I'll drink all my greens. I have a big container of nutrient-dense powdered greens; I just add water and drink it. It has just about everything you need. I also make smoothies with similar ingredients. I put some pineapple and strawberries in there with spinach and almond milk.

In my refrigerator you'll always find a lot of fruit, and pineapple is my favorite. Pineapple, grapes, and some good watermelon are the best. You'll also find plenty of kale, spinach, and beets—for meals and for juices.

Before games I have granola in almond milk with cinnamon because it's filling

FULL NAME: Giancarlo Cruz-Michael Stanton

HEIGHT/WEIGHT: 6'6", 245 lbs

BORN: November 8, 1989, in Panorama City, CA

POSITION: Right fielder

DRAFT: Drafted by the Florida Marlins in the 2nd round of the 2007 MLB Draft

HIGH SCHOOL: Notre Dame High School (Sherman Oaks, CA)

AWARDS AND RECOGNITION: 4x NL All-Star; 2017 NL MVP; 2017 NL RBI leader; 2x NL Silver Slugger Award; 2x Hank Aaron Award; 2016 Home Run Derby Champion; 2x NL home run leader

but not heavy. The cinnamon is great. It adds a little sweetness without the sugar.

I made a huge transition recently to eating mainly fish and eliminating meat. My body doesn't necessarily respond poorly to meat, and I loved eating it, but I much prefer the long-term benefit to my body from eating fish. I could eat salmon every day—either grilled or baked. Baked is probably my favorite because I like that texture.

Besides eating smart, I also practice hot yoga—I love the challenge of lengthening my body and strengthening my mind. I practice yoga mostly in the off-season. It's important to be limber and to balance strength. And it's hard! I go to a studio because I like being next to people who do it all the time. I'm amazed by other yogis who barely even sweat, while I'm sweating buckets. And I meditate after. The instructor says to think about the reasons for being here and all that, and to just let it all out. So, when difficulty and adversity come into my life, such as not having a good game, I try to put it in perspective and think about people who have it way more difficult in life than I do. I don't take anything for granted, and I know I have to keep working hard. I also know when I gotta chill out, and I understand that some things are not the end-all-be-all.

KHICHADI/YOGI BOWL

SERVES: 2 // **PREP:** *15 minutes, plus 1½ to 12 hours soaking time for rice* //
COOK: *55 minutes*

Not to be confused with Yogi Berra, this yogi bowl originated in India. *khichadi* ("food from the gods") is the ultimate wellness food. Easily digestible, it gives your body a break and helps it detox. It offers a great base of lentils and brown rice with aromatic spices. Take a deep breath, exhale, and savor every bite.

1½ teaspoons coconut oil

¼ cup finely chopped onion

1 tablespoon grated peeled ginger root

1 tablespoon grated garlic

½ teaspoon ground coriander

½ teaspoon ground cumin

¼ teaspoon crushed red pepper flakes

½ cup chopped tomato

¼ cup split red lentils

¼ cup short-grain brown rice, soaked

Salt

2 tablespoons chopped fresh cilantro, for serving

NOTE: Split red lentils do not require soaking.

1. In a medium saucepan, heat the oil over medium heat. Add the onion and cook until golden brown, stirring frequently, about 3 minutes. Stir in the ginger, garlic, coriander, cumin, and red pepper flakes and cook, stirring frequently, for 30 seconds.

2. Add the tomato, lentils, rice, and 2 cups water and reduce the heat to low. Simmer, covered, for 50 minutes to 1 hour, until smooth and creamy.

3. Season with salt to taste and divide between 2 bowls. Top with cilantro.

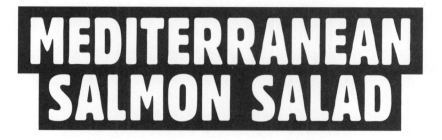

MEDITERRANEAN SALMON SALAD

SERVES: *2* // **PREP:** *15 minutes* // **COOK:** *10 minutes*

Wild salmon is Giancarlo Stanton's favorite fish because of its satisfying taste and healthful omega-3s. Whether you make it for lunch or as an easy weeknight dinner, it's a guaranteed home run.

2 (4-ounce) skin-on wild salmon fillets

1½ cups (½-inch) diced zucchini

3 tablespoons chopped fresh flat-leaf parsley

2 tablespoons chopped fresh dill

2 tablespoons fresh lemon juice

2 tablespoons extra-virgin olive oil

Salt and freshly ground pepper

3 cups baby spinach

½ ripe avocado, sliced

1 tablespoon hemp hearts

1. In a medium saucepan, bring 1 inch of water to a low simmer. Add the salmon, cover, and cook the fish until it is opaque in the center, 5 to 7 minutes, depending on thickness. Using a slotted spoon, transfer to a plate, lift off the skin, and let the salmon cool.

2. In a large bowl, combine the zucchini, parsley, dill, lemon juice, and oil. Gently break the salmon into chunks and carefully fold it into the mixture. Season with salt and pepper to taste.

3. Arrange a bed of spinach in 2 wide salad bowls. Place the salmon mixture on top. Lay half the avocado slices over each salad and sprinkle with the hemp hearts.

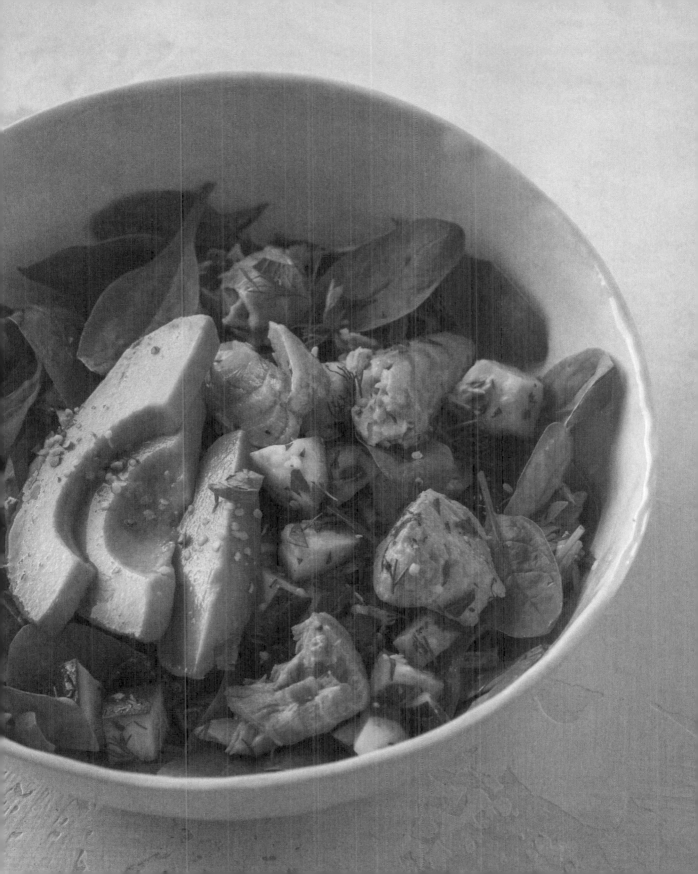

CINNAMON ALMOND FIG BARS

MAKES: *8 bars* // **PREP:** *15 minutes, plus 1 hour to chill* // **COOK:** *10 minutes*

This deliciously nutty and naturally sweet energy bar (pictured on page 23) will help satisfy your next snackable moment. Refrigerated individually wrapped bars are an easy grab-and-go treat.

¾ cup almonds

½ cup walnuts

1 cup dried black Mission figs, stems removed, chopped

½ cup dates, pitted and chopped

1 tablespoon ground cinnamon

1. Preheat the oven to 375°F.

2. Arrange the almonds and walnuts in a single layer on a baking sheet and toast for 7 to 9 minutes, until they just start to brown. Let cool before transferring to a food processor, then pulse until coarsely ground (you should have about 1¼ cups). Put the nuts in a large bowl.

2. Put the figs and dates in the food processor and blend, scraping down the sides, until a paste forms, about 2 minutes. Add the paste and cinnamon to the bowl with the nuts and use your hands to knead the ingredients into a dough.

3. On a parchment-lined sheet pan, press the dough with your hands into a 4 x 4-inch square and refrigerate for 1 hour. Cut into 8 bars (1 x 2 inches). Wrapped in wax paper in a sealed plastic bag or airtight container and refrigerated, the bars will keep for about 3 months.

ARUGULA SALAD

with Baked Wild Salmon and Cilantro Garlic Sauce

SERVES: *2* // **PREP:** *15 minutes* // **COOK:** *15 minutes*

The jicama adds a refreshing burst of sweetness, and the garlic sauce with cilantro provides a wonderful tangy topping to the salmon.

2 (¼-inch-thick) slices of red onion

2 teaspoons coconut oil, melted

2 (4-ounce) skin-on wild salmon fillets, deboned

Salt and freshly ground pepper

3 cups baby arugula

½ cup thinly shaved peeled jicama

1 tablespoon champagne vinegar

1 tablespoon extra-virgin olive oil

2 tablespoons Pickled Jalapeños (recipe follows on page 213)

2 tablespoons Cilantro Garlic Sauce (recipe follows on page 213)

1. Preheat the broiler to high and set a rack 6 inches from the heat source.

2. Arrange the onion in a single layer on a small baking sheet and toss with 1 teaspoon of the coconut oil. Broil, turning the slices halfway through, until golden brown, 4 to 5 minutes total. Transfer the onion to a cutting board and coarsely chop (you should have about ¼ cup).

3. Preheat the oven to 400°F.

4. Rub the salmon with the remaining 1 teaspoon coconut oil and season with salt and pepper to taste. Bake, skin-side down, for 7 to 10 minutes, depending on thickness, until opaque and firm to the touch.

5. In a medium bowl, combine the arugula, jicama, red onion, champagne vinegar, olive oil, and pickled jalapeños. Season with salt and pepper to taste.

6. Divide the salad between 2 bowls. Top each salad with a salmon fillet and a dollop of cilantro garlic sauce.

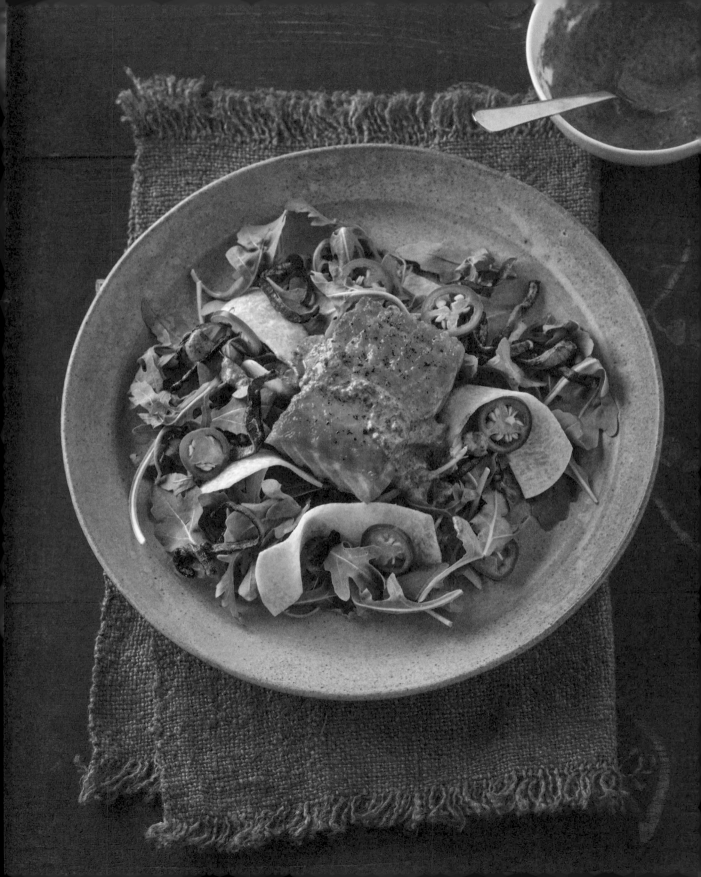

PICKLED JALAPEÑOS

SERVES: *2* // **PREP:** *5 minutes, plus 1 hour marinating time* // **COOK:** *5 minutes*

2 tablespoons white wine vinegar

2 tablespoons unseasoned rice wine vinegar

½ teaspoon coconut sugar

½ teaspoon salt

⅓ cup sliced jalapeños (see Note)

1. In a saucepan over medium heat, bring ¾ cup water, both vinegars, sugar, and salt to a boil. Reduce the heat to low, and then simmer for 2 minutes. Put the jalapeños in a large heatproof glass container (like a mason jar). Pour the hot liquid over the jalapeños. Let stand for at least 1 hour.

2. Once they've cooled to room temperature, store the jalapeños in the refrigerator in an airtight container for up to 4 weeks.

Note: For a milder level of heat, boil the jalapeños in water for 5 minutes and drain them before pickling.

CILANTRO GARLIC SAUCE

SERVES: *2* // **PREP:** *10 minutes*

2 cups packed fresh cilantro sprigs (about 1 bunch)

4 small garlic cloves, smashed

1 tablespoon fresh lime juice

¼ cup extra-virgin olive oil

¼ teaspoon salt

In a high-powered blender, combine all of the ingredients and process until smooth.

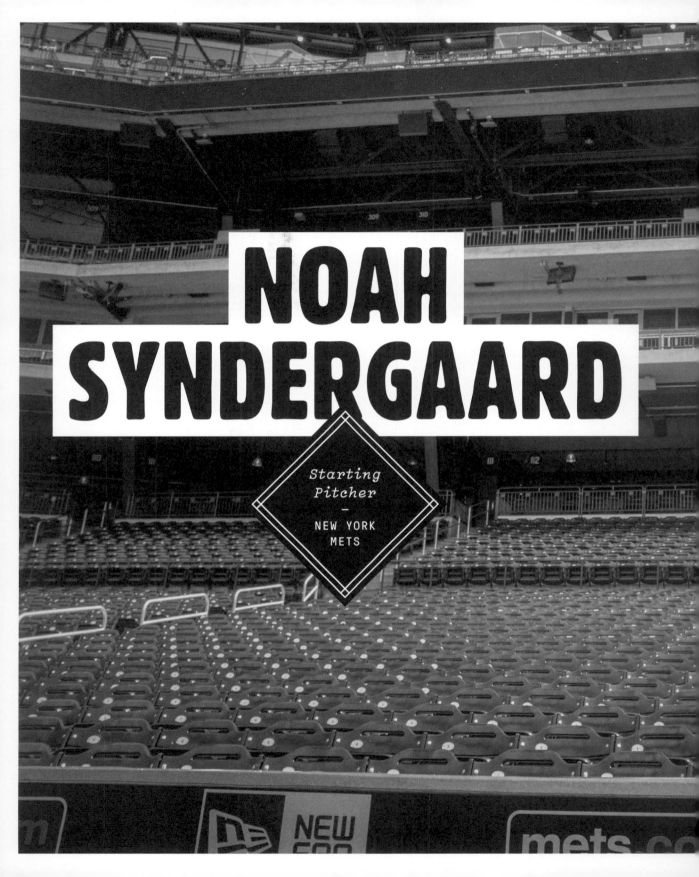

NOAH SYNDERGAARD

Starting
Pitcher
–
NEW YORK
METS

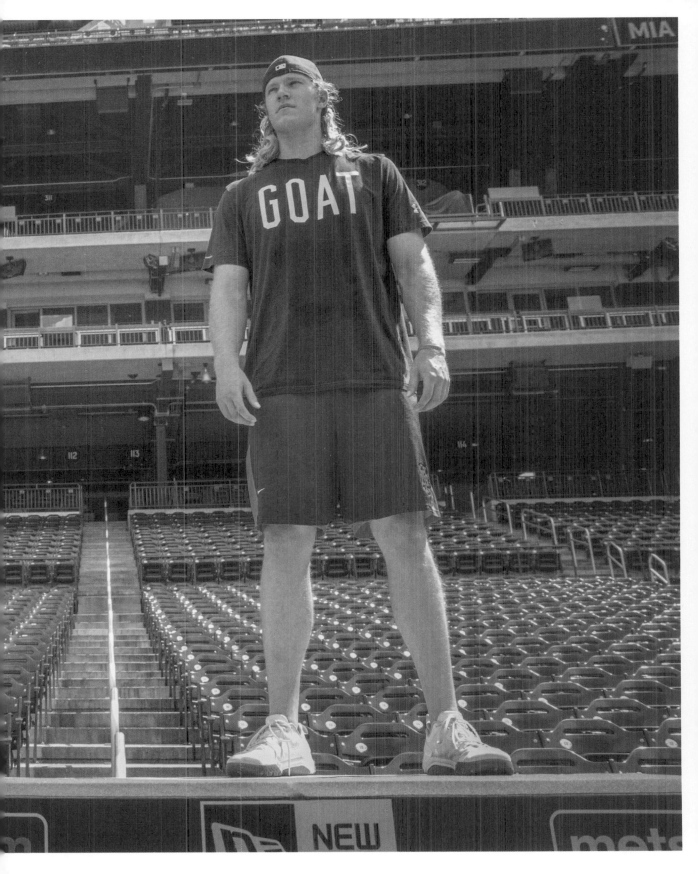

I want to go out there on the field each day and feel my absolute best, and good nutrition makes that possible. We're professional athletes, and we should take care of our bodies. At the end of the day if I don't reach my goals in my career, at least I can say that I gave it my all and covered all the bases. I want to play the game for a long time, and I don't want to wait until it's too late to jump on board with healthy eating.

I feel really good—optimistic and positive—coming to the ballpark. I believe my eating habits connect to my performance on the mound because I wake up every day and have a bunch of energy.

My breakfast today was almond butter protein pancakes with chicken sausage and fruit on the side. For lunch, I had Thai grilled chicken with quinoa and a mango-avocado salsa. I'm getting to that point where every city I travel to during the season is going to be set up with food made by a chef. For on-the-road games, my nutritionist sends me a list of all the healthy restaurants and juice bars in that particular city, or arranges to have a chef send healthy meals to my hotel. My dinner last night was braised beef short ribs with a sweet potato puree and Brussels

FULL NAME: Noah Seth Syndergaard

HEIGHT/WEIGHT: 6'6", 240 lbs

POSITION: Pitcher

BORN: August 29, 1992, in Mansfield, TX

DRAFT: Drafted by the Toronto Blue Jays in the 1st round (38th) of the 2010 MLB Draft

HIGH SCHOOL: Legacy High School (Mansfield, TX)

AWARDS AND RECOGNITION: 2016 NL All-Star

sprouts. Tonight it's something similar, but I'll have roasted cauliflower and green beans with it.

I follow a set structure for my meals, so that when I'm on the field, I can maximize my performance based on what I've eaten throughout the day. The only thing that changes is I'll carbo-load for lunch the day before I pitch. That means eating something heavier, like a sweet potato or another good complex carb.

In my refrigerator you'll always find essential healthy snacks like protein cookies, chia seed bars, and a lot of water and juices. I'm also a big fan of roasted cauliflower now, so I usually have cauliflower on hand too.

My favorite fresh juice is a combination of beet, carrot, pear, apple, pineapple, and ginger—I bought a juicer, and I'm juicing every day. I go to the grocery store and pick up a bunch of beets and juice anything and everything, like carrots, apple, peppers, kale, Swiss chard, spinach—even jalapeños, but just a small slice to give a little kick. I did a three-day juice cleanse in the off-season to give my digestive system a break. It wasn't anything structured, and I could have smoothies too. I noticed my energy levels just skyrocketed.

"I follow a set structure for my meals, so that when I'm on the field, I can maximize my performance based on what I've eaten throughout the day. The only thing that changes is I'll carbo-load for lunch the day before I pitch. That means eating something heavier, like a sweet potato or another good complex carb."

I also like smoothies—my favorite includes blueberries, dates, almond milk, coconut nectar, coconut meat, and all kinds of good stuff. I prefer fresh juices instead of smoothies, but that one's pretty good. To help speed muscle recovery after a tough workout, I take a lot of turmeric and drink tart cherry juice as an anti-inflammatory.

My former former teammate Curtis Granderson gave me a great piece of advice. He said, "When you wake up every day, you have a choice to be positive." He's the nicest guy you'll ever meet. He's always in a good mood. Even when he has a bad game, he's never angry. I try to be positive every day.

CHICKEN BURGER
with Roasted Cauliflower

SERVES: *2* // **PREP:** *10 minutes* // **COOK:** *10 minutes*

Swap your hamburger and fries for this tasty chicken burger with a side of roasted cauliflower and greens. It's a nourishing win-win.

1 tablespoon plus 1 teaspoon coconut oil

¼ cup minced shallots

8 ounces ground chicken (white and dark meat)

⅓ cup almond flour

1½ teaspoons fresh lemon juice

½ teaspoon salt

½ teaspoon ground turmeric

¼ teaspoon freshly ground pepper

Roasted Cauliflower and Greens (recipe follows)

1. In a small skillet over medium heat, heat 1 teaspoon of the oil. Add the shallots and cook, stirring occasionally, until golden brown, about 2 minutes. Let cool.

2. In a medium bowl, mix the chicken, flour, lemon juice, salt, turmeric, pepper, and cooled shallots until well combined.

3. Shape into 4 (3 x ⅓-inch) patties (rubbing a dab of oil on your palms will help prevent the meat from sticking). Heat the remaining 1 tablespoon oil in a medium nonstick skillet over medium heat. Cook the burgers, adjusting the heat as necessary, until golden brown on both sides and cooked through, 6 to 7 minutes total. Serve with roasted cauliflower and greens.

ROASTED CAULIFLOWER AND GREENS

SERVES: *2* // **PREP:** *15 minutes* // **COOK:** *15 minutes*

3 cups cauliflower florets

1 tablespoon coconut oil, melted

Pinch of cayenne

1½ cups chopped dinosaur kale, tough ribs removed first

Salt and freshly ground black pepper

1. Preheat the oven to 425°F.

2. In a medium bowl, toss the cauliflower with the oil and cayenne. Arrange in a single layer on a baking sheet and roast until just tender, about 10 minutes.

3. Remove the baking sheet from the oven and, using tongs, fold the kale in with the cauliflower. Return to the oven and continue to roast for 1 to 2 minutes, until the kale is slightly wilted. Season with salt and pepper to taste.

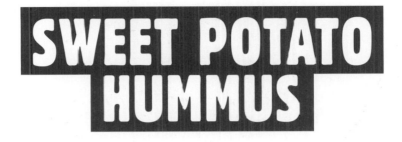

SWEET POTATO HUMMUS

SERVES: *4* // **PREP:** *5 minutes* // **COOK:** *50 minutes*

Change up chickpea hummus for a creamier sweet potato version. The cumin gives an added depth of gorgeous flavor.

1 large sweet potato
1 teaspoon coconut oil
1 tablespoon finely chopped garlic
2 tablespoons extra-virgin olive oil
1½ tablespoons fresh lemon juice
1 tablespoon tahini
¾ teaspoon ground cumin
Salt

1. Preheat the oven to 375°F.

2. Place the sweet potato on a small baking sheet and bake until soft, 40 to 45 minutes. When cool enough to handle, remove the skin and coarsely chop. You should have about 2 cups.

3. In a small skillet, melt the coconut oil over medium heat. Add the garlic and cook, stirring, until golden brown, about 1 minute. In a high-powered blender, combine the garlic, sweet potato, olive oil, lemon juice, tahini, and cumin and process until smooth. Season with salt to taste.

4. Serve as a dip for raw veggies such as carrots, cucumber, celery, and radishes.

SHORT RIBS

with Green Beans, Brussels Sprouts, and Ginger

SERVES: *4* // **PREP:** *25 minutes* // **COOK:** *4 hours*

You'll flip over these short ribs. A thick and flavorful sauce is key in this recipe, so opt for a natural beef stock to achieve the right consistency. The subtle-tasting gingered green veggies complete this gratifying meal.

2 pounds bone-in short ribs

¼ teaspoon salt, plus more to taste

¼ teaspoon freshly ground pepper, plus more to taste

2 tablespoons coconut oil

1 cup chopped onion

1 cup chopped celery

½ cup chopped carrot

10 small garlic cloves

1 stalk lemongrass, tough outer layers removed, chopped

1 tablespoon tomato paste

2 quarts beef stock

4 sprigs fresh rosemary

2 bay leaves

Green Beans and Brussels Sprouts with Ginger (recipe follows on page 222)

1. Preheat the oven to 350°F.

2. Season the ribs with ¼ teaspoon each salt and pepper. In a heavy ovenproof 5-quart pot, heat the oil over high heat until hot but not smoking. Brown the ribs on all sides until deep golden brown, about 10 minutes total. Transfer the ribs to a plate.

3. Reduce the heat to medium-high and add the onion, celery, carrot, garlic, and lemongrass. Cook, stirring occasionally, until golden brown, 6 to 8 minutes. Stir in the tomato paste and cook, stirring constantly, for 2 minutes.

4. Add the stock, rosemary, bay leaves, and browned ribs with any juices and bring just to a boil. Cover tightly and bake in the middle of oven for 3 to 3½ hours, until fork-tender.

5. Transfer the meat and bones to a plate. On top of the stove, bring the liquid to a boil. Simmer until reduced to 2½ to 3 cups, about 30 minutes. Strain the sauce through a fine-mesh sieve and season with more salt and pepper, if desired. Remove excess fat with a spoon.

6. Once the meat has cooled, cut away the fat and connective tissue near the bone and slice. Pour the sauce on top of the meat.

7. Serve with the green beans and Brussels sprouts.

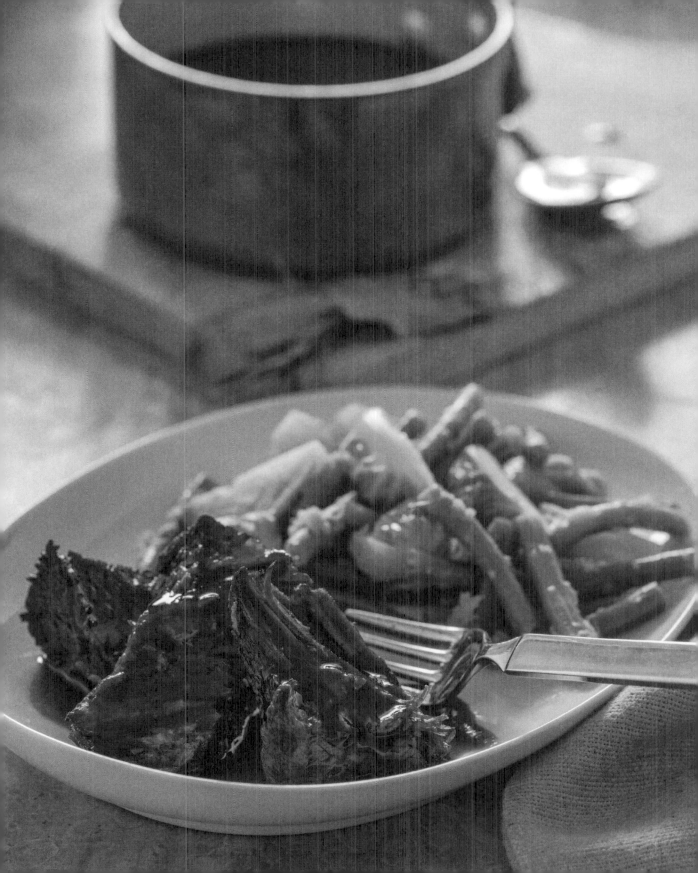

GREEN BEANS AND BRUSSELS SPROUTS WITH GINGER

SERVES: *4* // **PREP:** *10 minutes* // **COOK:** *5 minutes*

1 tablespoon coconut oil

2 tablespoons finely chopped yellow onion

1 tablespoon grated ginger

1½ cups halved trimmed green beans

1½ cups quartered Brussels sprouts

Salt and freshly ground pepper

1. In a medium saucepan over medium heat, heat the oil. Add the onion and ginger and cook, stirring constantly, until golden brown, about 2 minutes.

2. Add the green beans, Brussels sprouts, and ½ cup water. Cover and steam the veggies until tender, about 3 minutes.

3. Remove from the heat and season with salt and pepper to taste.

CHERRY CHIA BARS

MAKES: *8 bars* // **PREP:** *10 minutes, plus 1 hour to chill*

Get fist-pumping energy with these delightful cherry power bars. Tiny chia seeds are packed with nutrients and potent micronutrients. When shopping for the dried Medjool dates, look for soft ones for the best texture.

1½ cups unsweetened dried dark cherries

1 cup pitted Medjool dates

¾ cup almonds

¾ cup pecans

3 tablespoons chia seeds

1½ teaspoons raw honey

1. Line a baking sheet with wax paper or parchment.

2. In a food processor, pulse the cherries, dates, almonds, pecans, and chia seeds until finely chopped, about 25 pulses. Add the honey and process for 2 to 3 minutes, until the mixture is nearly smooth and starts to come together into a ball. Transfer the mixture to the lined baking sheet, scraping out the processor bowl with a rubber spatula, if needed. With your hands, shape the mixture into a 6 x 6 x 1-inch square.

3. Refrigerate for 1 hour. With a sharp knife, trim the square and cut into 8 (3 x 1½-inch) bars. Wrap individually in wax paper and store in the fridge in a sealed plastic bag or airtight container. The bars will keep for about 3 months.

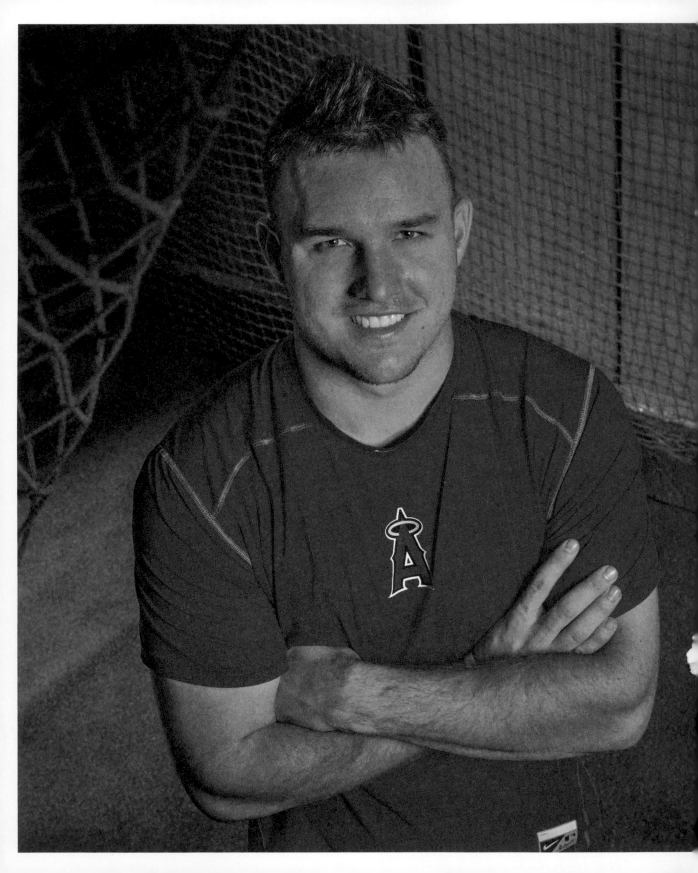

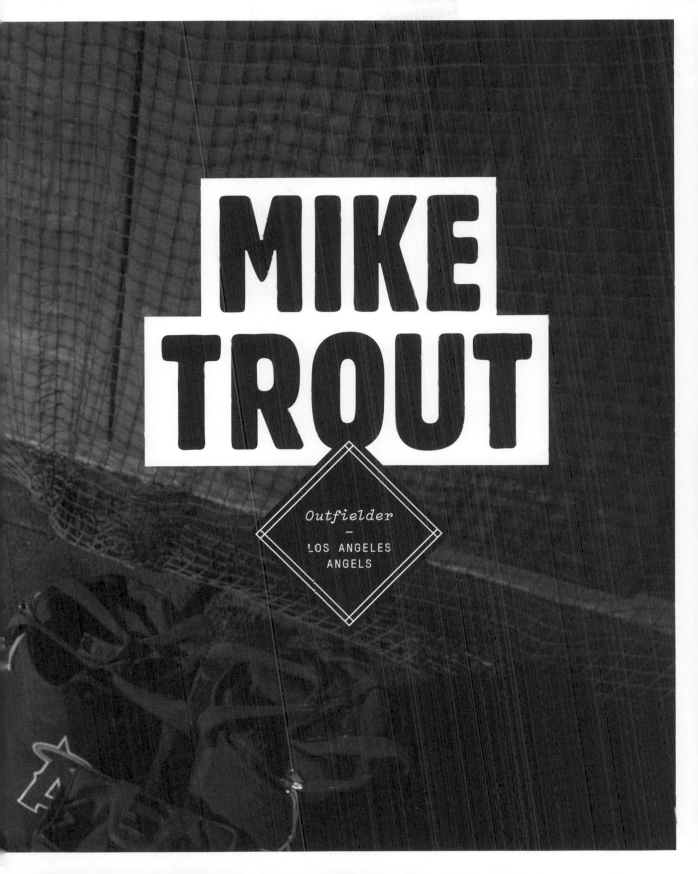

MIKE TROUT

Outfielder
—
LOS ANGELES
ANGELS

My morning routine varies and my lifestyle is different from most people's because of baseball. When we play a night game, I get home at midnight or one in the morning. After I get home, I'll go right to bed. I wake up around 11 or 11:30, so my breakfast is everyone else's lunch.

For lunch I really like a salad with lots of greens and a protein like chicken or steak. Ask anyone in the clubhouse how I prepare for a game, they'll tell you that I'm a big chicken and beef guy. And I love pickles. In my refrigerator, you'll always find the ingredients to make salads and a simple balsamic vinaigrette.

I try to drink a fresh juice once a day—it's a good balance for me because I eat a lot of protein and I have to get my vegetables in there too. My favorite fresh juice is a mix of vegetable and fruit. I like kale, ginger, carrots, apples, and oranges. I'm a big beets guy. I have this for lunch or breakfast. Fresh juices are the biggest things now in our clubhouse.

Dinner is often lighter than lunch because our games end so late. I always include asparagus, a side salad, and a protein, like a steak. I also love seafood like crab, lobster, and tuna, and I just started to like sushi.

I recently discovered that I like ginger; it's good for you and fights inflammation. It's a tough taste to handle at first, but once you get used to it, it's really good. I add it to my fresh juices.

I always try to stay hydrated when I'm working out or playing in order to keep my energy up. I know when my body is feeling good and when it's not. I know if I'm sluggish or slow that day or week, how my body reacts to certain foods. When you put something in your body, you should know how it makes you feel. If your reaction afterward is that you're sluggish, then you know it was connected to something you ate. For me, it's important to be my best.

FULL NAME: Michael Nelson Trout

HEIGHT/WEIGHT: 6'2", 235 lbs

BORN: August 7, 1991, in Vineland, NJ

POSITION: Centerfielder

DRAFT: Drafted by the Los Angeles Angels of Anaheim in the 1st round (25th) of the 2009 MLB Draft

HIGH SCHOOL: Millville Senior High School (Millville, NJ)

AWARDS AND RECOGNITION: 7x AL All-Star; 2x AL MVP; 2012 AL ROY; 6x AL Silver Slugger Award; 2014 AL Hank Aaron Award; 2014 AL RBI leader; 2012 AL stolen base leader; 2012 30-30 club; hit for the cycle on May 21, 2013

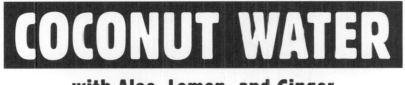

COCONUT WATER

with Aloe, Lemon, and Ginger

SERVES: *1* // **PREP:** *5 minutes*

The aloe helps to maintain the proper balance of alkalinity in your body. Use aloe water, not aloe juice, when making this deliciously revitalizing drink.

1 cup chilled aloe water
1 cup chilled raw coconut water
½ lemon, sliced
1-inch piece of ginger root, sliced

Combine all the ingredients in a jar and infuse in the refrigerator for a minimum of 12 hours. This drink will keep, refrigerated, for up to 4 days. Strain into glasses before serving.

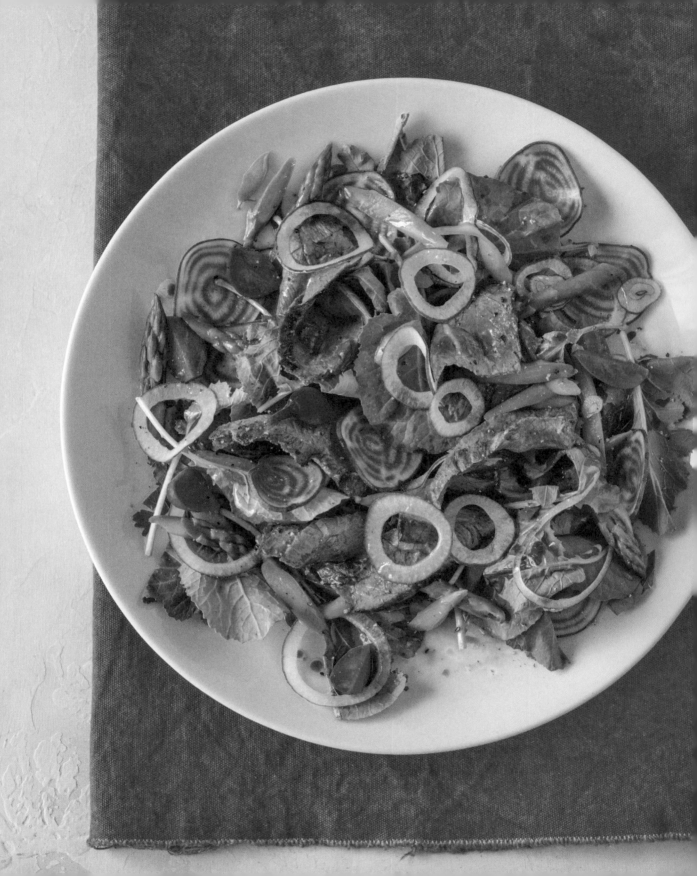

SKIRT STEAK SALAD

with Pickled Radishes

SERVES: *2* // **PREP:** *25 minutes* // **COOK:** *5 minutes*

Mike Trout enjoys eating a really good steak just as much as he enjoys eating a really good salad, so why not put the two together? The pickled radishes, veggies, and vinaigrette further enhance the robust steak flavors.

1½ cups thinly sliced asparagus

8 ounces grass-fed skirt steak, trimmed of excess fat

½ teaspoon smoked salt

¼ teaspoon freshly ground pepper

1½ teaspoons coconut oil

3 cups baby kale

½ cup chopped fresh flat-leaf parsley

½ cup thinly shaved peeled raw beets, such as Chioggia (also called candy stripe)

¼ cup thinly shaved red onion

2 tablespoons Balsamic Vinaigrette (recipe follows on page 230)

¼ cup Pickled Radishes (recipe follows on page 230)

1. In a saucepan fitted with a steamer basket, bring 1 inch of water to a boil. Put the asparagus in the basket, cover, and steam for 30 seconds. Remove the basket and let the asparagus cool while you cook the steak.

2. Rub the steak with the smoked salt and pepper. Heat the oil in a cast-iron skillet over medium-high heat until hot but not smoking. Add the steak and once it starts to brown, reduce the heat to medium; continue to sear on both sides to the desired doneness, 2 to 3 minutes per side for medium. (A skirt steak is best at medium rare to medium. Otherwise it can be tough and chewy.) Let the steak rest for 5 minutes before slicing thinly against the grain.

3. In a medium bowl, combine the kale, reserved asparagus, parsley, beets, and red onion. Fold in the balsamic vinaigrette and divide between 2 salad bowls. Add half of the pickled radishes to each bowl and top with steak.

BALSAMIC VINAIGRETTE

SERVES: *2* // **PREP:** *5 minutes*

2 tablespoons balsamic vinegar
⅓ cup extra-virgin olive oil
Salt and freshly ground pepper

Pour the vinegar into a small bowl. Add the oil in a slow stream, whisking constantly. Season with salt and pepper to taste.

PICKLED RADISHES

SERVES: *2* // **PREP:** *5 minutes, plus 1 hour marinating time* // **COOK:** *5 minutes*

1 cup radishes, trimmed and quartered
2 tablespoons white wine vinegar
2 tablespoons cider vinegar
¼ teaspoon black peppercorns
⅛ teaspoon salt
1 sprig fresh thyme

1. In a small saucepan over medium heat, combine 1/2 cup water, both vinegars, peppercorns, salt, and thyme and cook for 2 minutes. Put the radishes in a heatproof glass container (like a mason jar). Pour the hot liquid over the radishes. Let stand for at least 1 hour.

2. Once they have cooled to room temperature, store the radishes in the refrigerator for up to 4 weeks.

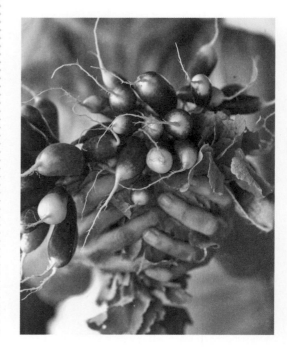

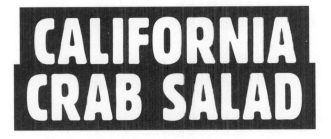

CALIFORNIA CRAB SALAD

SERVES: 2 // **PREP:** 1 hour 15 minutes

This salad is brimming with fresh flavors in every bite. Making the gorgeous cherry tomato dressing is a cinch. Don't forget the pea sprouts, which are packed with nutrients and are a snap to add to any dish.

2 cups thinly sliced bok choy or arugula

½ cup pea sprouts

2 tablespoons sprouted lentils (optional)

½ cup Pickled Cucumbers (recipe follows on page 233)

4 ounces jumbo lump crabmeat, tough pieces of cartilage removed

Salt and freshly ground black pepper

½ cup Roasted Cherry Tomato Dressing (recipe follows on page 233)

1. In a medium bowl, combine the bok choy, sprouts, lentils (if using), and pickled cucumbers. Fold in the crabmeat and season with salt and pepper to taste.

2. Divide between 2 bowls and spoon some of the tomato dressing evenly over each salad.

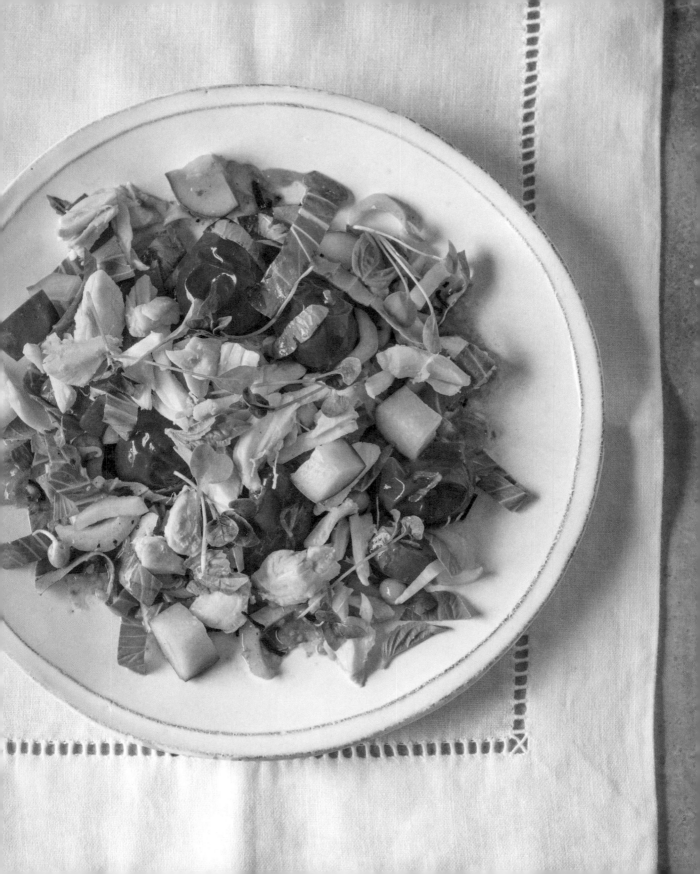

PICKLED CUCUMBERS

SERVES: *2* // **PREP:** *10 minutes, plus 1 hour marinating time* // **COOK:** *5 minutes*

3 tablespoons unseasoned rice wine vinegar

2 tablespoons cider vinegar

1 garlic clove, smashed

¼ teaspoon black peppercorns

⅛ teaspoon salt

1 cup diced cucumbers, unpeeled

1. In a small saucepan, bring ½ cup water, both vinegars, garlic, peppercorns, and salt to a boil. Reduce the heat to medium-low and simmer for 3 minutes. Put the diced cucumber in a heatproof glass container (like a mason jar) big enough to hold the liquid and strain the hot liquid over the cucumbers. Let stand at room temperature for at least 1 hour.

2. Once the cucumbers have cooled, cover tightly and refrigerate for up to 4 weeks.

ROASTED CHERRY TOMATO DRESSING

SERVES: *2* // **PREP:** *10 minutes* // **COOK:** *15 minutes*

1 cup cherry tomatoes

1 tablespoon thinly sliced shallot

½ teaspoon coconut oil, melted

Salt and freshly ground pepper

1½ tablespoons fresh lemon juice

1½ tablespoons extra-virgin olive oil

1 tablespoon torn basil

1. Preheat the broiler.

2. Combine the tomatoes, shallot, coconut oil, and salt and pepper to taste on a baking sheet. Broil until the tomatoes are just starting to blister, about 6 minutes.

3. Transfer the tomatoes to a small bowl and toss with the lemon juice, olive oil, and basil. Season with salt and pepper to taste.

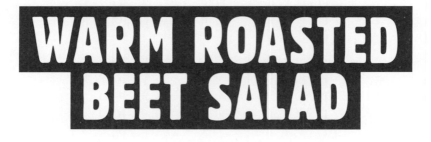

WARM ROASTED BEET SALAD

SERVES: *2* // **PREP:** *15 minutes* // **COOK:** *1 hour*

This straightforward salad is chock-full of plant protein, complex carbs, and healthy fats. A plant-based "cheese" is a great healthy alternative to dairy and should contain just a few simple ingredients. Choose one that is nut-based, like cashew, but also contains nutritional yeast, probiotics, and lemon juice.

2 tablespoons pistachios

4 medium beets, red or yellow or a combination, stems trimmed to 1 inch

½ teaspoon coconut oil, melted

2 teaspoons vinegar (cider for yellow beets, red wine for red beets)

2 teaspoons extra-virgin olive oil

Salt and freshly ground pepper

3 cups baby arugula or beet greens

2 tablespoons Balsamic Vinaigrette (page 230)

2 tablespoons soft cashew cheese

1. Preheat the oven to 375°F.

2. Arrange the pistachios in a single layer on a baking sheet and roast for 7 minutes, until lightly browned. Set the nuts aside until cool enough to handle, then chop.

3. Meanwhile, put the beets in a small baking dish and toss with the coconut oil. Cover the dish with foil and roast the beets until tender, 50 to 90 minutes, depending on their size. Insert a wooden skewer into the thickest part of the beets periodically. The skewer will slide in easily when the beets are done. When the beets are cool enough to handle, use a paper towel to peel them. Do not rinse. (Use gloves or slide your hands into plastic sandwich bags for red beets as they will stain your hands.)

4. Cut the warm beets into wedges. Immediately put into a medium bowl and toss with the vinegar, olive oil, and salt and pepper to taste.

5. Divide the arugula between 2 salad bowls. (If you have fresh greens from the beets, you can use those instead. Trim the stems, and reserve for another use, then slice the leaves.) Drizzle balsamic vinaigrette over the greens. Add the dressed beets.

6. Roll the cheese into 4 balls and add 2 to each salad. Top with the toasted pistachios. Serve immediately.

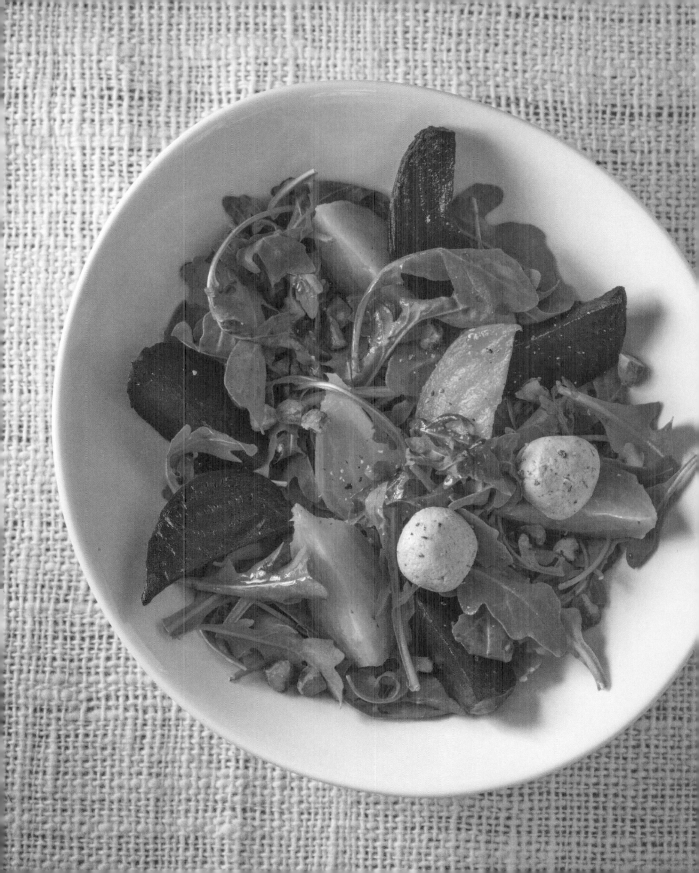

ACKNOWLEDGMENTS

A heartfelt thank-you to the many people who supported my book journey. I could not have accomplished my goal without the support of Major League Baseball (MLB) and especially Commissioner Robert Manfred, whose passion for the game is unparalleled.

I would also like to thank the Major League Baseball Players Association executive director, Tony Clark.

And to Tony Petitti and Dan Halem, and many of the MLB and MLBPA folks for their guidance and enthusiasm, especially Ethan Orlinsky (MLB) and Tim Slavin (MLBPA).

I am beyond grateful to the MLB teams and players who graciously participated, and to the following people who were so helpful along the way:

Elizabeth Ayers
Mike Berger
Scott Boras
Jessica Carroll
Tony Carullo
Brian Cashman
Peter Chase
Matt Chisholm
Adam Chodzko
Manny Colón
Amanda Comak
Claude Delorme
Gene Dias

Fredi González
Kevin Gregg
Brad Hainje
Jay Horowitz
Kristen Hudak
Rock Hughes
Joe Jareck
Eric Kay
Jeff King
Simon Lusky
Don Mattingly
Beth McConville
Warren Miller

Jenny Perez
Mike Rizzo
Matt Roebuck
John Silverman
Miguel Solis
Jay Stenhouse

Bart Swain
Rick Vaughn
Aileen Villarreal
Joel Wolfe
Jason Zillo
Marcello Zito

Thank you to Jamie Banks, David Corporan, Yvette Freixas, and John Tavarez.

Thank you, Green Thumb Farmstand (especially Jo Halsey and Debbie Lehman) and Seven Ponds Farmstand.

Thank you to Rodale Books and Mark Weinstein for first seeing the potential in my idea; and to my agent, Susan Ginsburg, for helping to turn my idea into a reality.

And to my editor, Alyse Diamond (who became a baseball fan during this process), and everyone at the Crown Publishing Group.

Thank you to Ben Fink and his photography team for all the beautiful shots; and to Chef Allen Campbell for his instrumental cooking expertise.

My dearest family and friends.

And my loving husband, Jeffrey, who now eats quinoa.

INDEX

Note: Page references in *italics* indicate photographs.

ABOUT THE AUTHORS

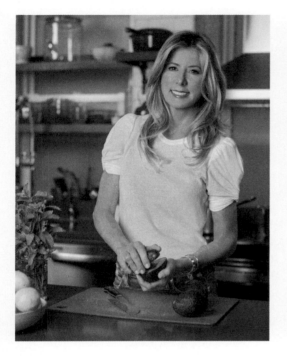

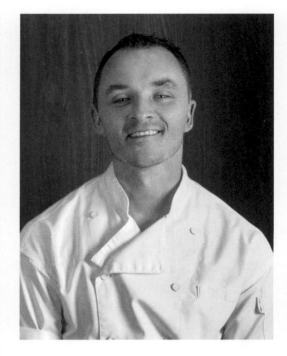

Julie Loria is the author of *Diamond Dishes*, her first book, which showcased stories and recipes from twenty top MLB players, including Derek Jeter, Albert Pujols, and Alex Rodriguez. She was born and raised a baseball fan, with a passion for food and cooking. She honed her culinary skills in Paris at the French cooking school La Cuisine de Marie-Blanche. She now lives in New York.

Allen Campbell is known as "the chef of peak performance." He was most recently the personal chef for the New England Patriots' star quarterback Tom Brady and his wife, Gisele Bündchen. With Tom, he coauthored the *TB12 Nutrition Manual*. Allen lives in Boston.